'A tremendous book. A perspective that needs to be heard.'
Oliver James, author, broadcaster and clinical psychologist.

'This is phenomenology—it reveals meaning through close observation, it's women's writing like Virginia Woolf.'
*Emerita Professor of Philosophy Eleanor Godway,
Central Connecticut State University.*

'A rollercoaster ride of emotion, courage, and political chicanery... I was held by the power of the narrative.'
Dave Marteau, former Head, HM Prison Service Drug Addiction Service.

'Captivating and most beautifully written.'
Jerome Carson, Professor of Psychology, University of Bolton.

'I was gripped... a great read. I would recommend the book to Prison Service colleagues.'
Tim Newell, former Governor, HM Prison Grendon.

'I nearly stood up... and clapped.'
Andrew Holden, film and TV scriptwriter.

The Prison Psychiatrist's Wife

Copyright © 2023 Sue Johnson.

All intellectual property and associated rights are hereby asserted and reserved by her in full compliance with UK and international law. No part of this book may be copied, reproduced, stored in any retrieval system or transmitted in any form or by any means without the prior written permission of the publishers to whom all such rights have been assigned worldwide.

The Foreword and images on p.xii are the copyright of Charles Bronson.

ISBN 978-1-914603-30-3 (Paperback)
ISBN 978-1-914603-31-0 (EPUB ebook)
ISBN 978-1-914603-32-7 (PDF ebook)

Published 2023 by Waterside Press Ltd
www.WatersidePress.co.uk

A catalogue record for this book can be obtained from the British Library.

Ebook *The Prison Psychiatrist's Wife* is available as an ebook including through library models.

Cover design Holly Rees www.hollyrees.co.uk © Waterside Press 2023.

The Prison Psychiatrist's Wife

Sue Johnson

Foreword Charles Bronson

WATERSIDE PRESS

The Prison Psychiatrist's Wife

Contents

Publisher's note *viii*
Acknowledgements *ix*
About the author *x*
Dedication *xi*

Foreword xiii
        The author of the Foreword *xiv*

Prologue xv

1 **The Beginnings** 17
        Eighteen months earlier *17*
        My first time inside a prison *19*
        A dinner party *24*
        The first week *26*

2 **The Strong Man** 31
        Shock and anger *34*
        Bob's increasing certainty *35*

3 **Early Days** 37
        We meet the CMO *38*
        The first murder threat *40*

4 **A Tea Party** 43
        Pink flowers and a piranha fish *44*
        They used to hang us here… *45*

5   **Trust and Change** 47
        Growing enthusiasm   *48*
        The first video-recording   *49*
        Pride   *53*
        And anger …   *55*

6   **The Man in the Blue Jumper** 57
        Darkness   *58*

7   **A Hopeful Time** 61
        The Big Man: my second encounter   *63*
        Persistence   *66*

8   **A Swimming Party** 69
        The Governors' Conference   *70*
        Early retirement   *74*

9   **A Barbecue** 77
        Spreading humanity   *77*
        Normality   *82*

10 **The Hospital Wing** 83
        Childhood influences   *84*
        Putting the videotapes on record   *86*

11 **The Guardian** 89
        Melanie   *89*
        Publication   *90*
        The backlash   *91*
        Finding a voice   *97*

12 **New Man on the Wing** 101
        Another painful video   *102*
        A huge sense of loss   *106*

13 **Grendon** 107
        An invitation *109*
        We join a therapy group *113*
        Signs of progress *116*
        Word spreads… *118*

14 **Prison Politics** 121
        A visit to the Home Office *121*
        The attack *122*
        A new Director-General of Prisons *123*
        Corridors of power *124*
        An outside view *127*

15 **Murder Threat** 131
        A puzzle to solve *131*
        Re-engagement *134*

16 **The Inspectorate Calls** 137
        The report *138*
        Bafflement *140*

17 **A Breaking Storm** 143
        An escape *143*
        Reaction of the new Home Secretary *145*
        Truth from nonsense *150*

18 **Resignation** 153
        Headline day *155*

19 **Panorama** 157
        Tom *157*
        Our demands and requirements *160*
        BBC studios *161*
        A date is set for the broadcast *163*

20 **The High Court** 165
    An injunction *165*
    An affidavit *167*
    The hearing *170*
    The judge's ruling *173*

21 **After-days** 177
    Final meeting *180*
    Farewell *181*

22 **After-shocks** 183
    One: The Big Man *183*
    Two: Baby of the wing *184*
    Three: The man in the blue jumper *185*
    An ending *187*

Epilogue *189*

Publisher's note

The views and opinions in this book are those of the author and not necessarily shared by the publisher. Whilst every effort has been made to ensure the fairness and accuracy of information contained in the text, readers should draw their own conclusions concerning the possibility of alternative views and explanations. The author has asked that we point out that with some individuals identifying details have been amended or changed to respect confidentiality.

Acknowledgements

Every writer needs someone at the beginning of their creative journey, and I was lucky to have two fine writers in Oliver James and Andrew Holden whose professional advice and opinion I respected. I sent the first four pages to Andrew and asked whether it was good enough writing, he said 'Yes!' Oliver read the first chapter and said, 'This is worth writing about, and you must continue.' This was the informed encouragement I needed. Once I'd completed the book, I was most fortunate to meet Professor Jerome Carson. He insisted that it needed to be published, which renewed my resolve to find a publisher.

I am also indebted to all my wonderful readers, who willingly read early drafts and gave me useful, accurate and encouraging feedback. Tim Newell, Dave Marteau, Harry Harris, Fiona Pearson, Marianne Johnson, Arabella Melville, Sam Winston, Eve Jackson, Mathew Scurfield, Eleanor Godway, Krys Pochin, Sue Haslam, Jean Payne, David Harrison, Robert Oliver, Katherine Oliver, Martin Johnson, Elsie Lyons, Millie Kieve, Stephen Hall, David George, Jill George, Liz Else, Jake Esman and Annabel Esman.

An especial thanks goes to Edwina Grosvenor for her longstanding interest and support in my particular story, and for her vision and charitable work in Social Justice.

I was extraordinarily blessed with the support of my family. My daughter Kate dropped everything to listen to my latest writing and offered insightful comment. My son-in-law Mark read instalments at night to my daughter Clare, providing me with early knowledge that what I was trying to do worked well.

A big thank you to my publishers, in particular Bryan, for his valuable understanding and expert and respectful editing. I couldn't have wished for better.

I also wish to thank 'Charlie' for his kind Foreword and the other prisoners I write about (mostly anonymously) for their courage.

Finally, fondest love and thanks to Bob, my life partner and husband whose unwavering vision fuelled this endeavour.

Sue Johnson, January 2023

The Prison Psychiatrist's Wife

About the author

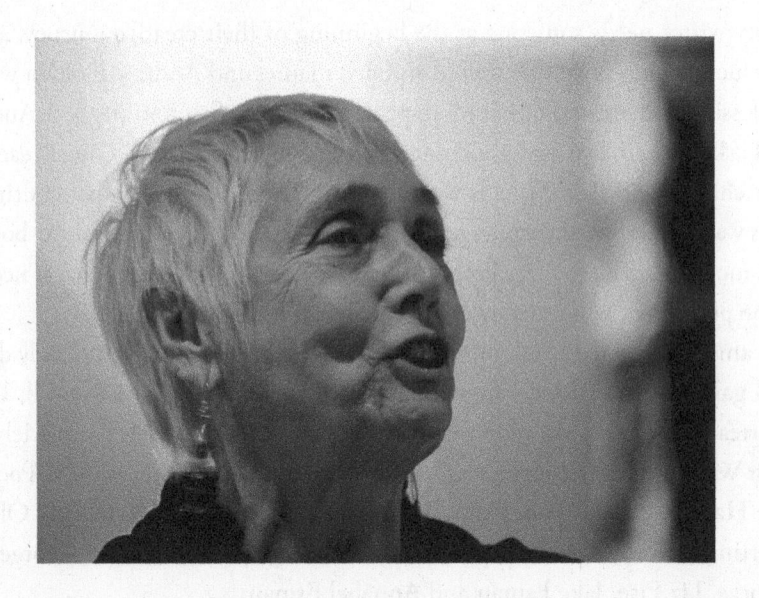

Sue Johnson now lives in central Manchester, delighting in her roof garden and entertaining friends and her large family. She is continuing her writing, thinking and research about Social Justice as well as working on her next book. Sue is about to celebrate her diamond wedding anniversary.

Photo: Justin Haslam

This book is dedicated to the late John Marriott for without his courage, humanity and vision this story would never have begun.

The Prison Psychiatrist's Wife

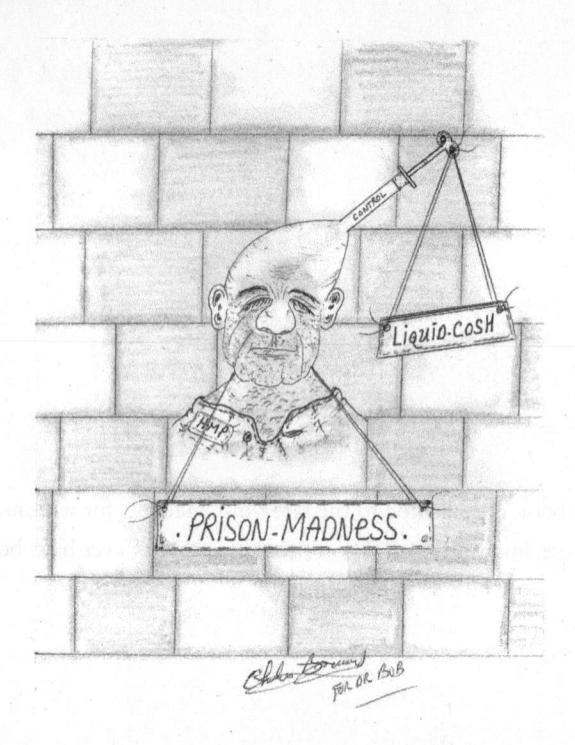

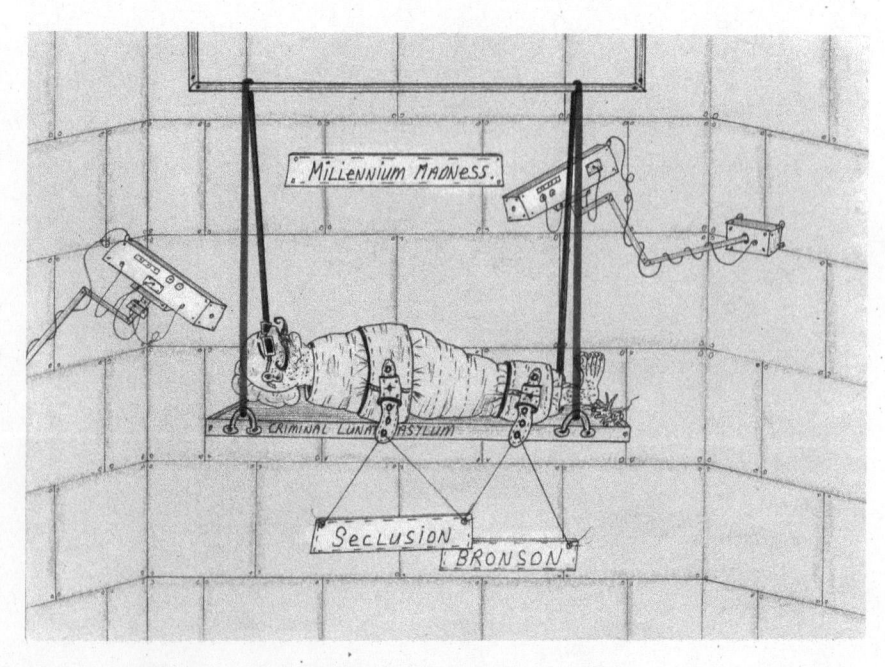

For Dr Bob from Charles Bronson

Foreword

Charles Bronson

Just copped Sue's manuscript. Very interesting read. I enjoyed it 'cos it's so unique. Simply as it's a wife on the outside with a story of how it feels for her husband to have such a crazy job. When 'Dr Bob' went to work, she never knew if he would come home with holes in him or in a zip up bag.

You must have been terrified Sue every morning at the breakfast table as Bob prepared for a day in madness. Always wondering if today would be his last! It sure took me to another world over the walls. Yours truly must have been pure insanity. Like being in a war zone (awaiting the phone call). My first wife has just had her book out, *The Truth, The Whole Truth and Nothing But The Truth*. All them years in the 1970s she never knew if her man would come home. Sadly, I never! She had to move on in life!

Men like Bob and John Marriott are a rare breed in my world. They earn respect. Sadly, it don't always work out. But nine times out of ten their way works. Why can't the system see it. What Bob achieved was magical. He helped so many and should be proud—and I've still to meet a better prison Governor than Mr Marriott.

'We the willing—led by the unknown—have been doing the impossible for the ungrateful for so long—with so little. Are we qualified to do anything at all?' A con called 'Big Andi' told me this in Parkhurst in the 1980s. He died in Bristol Jail in the 1990s. His whole life was violence, even his ending was violence. I reckon Bob could have helped him.

I've read so many books over the decades I've been in jail, from crime to cowboys, but I do enjoy a good autobiography. Sue's story I can honestly say is mind-provoking and a brilliant read. It would make a great movie or TV play. Films, books, plays on jails, asylums mostly portray convicts as lunatics. Your book balances it up. How the wife/partner/family outside feel about their stressful survival. And let's face it a max secure jail can and does often explode into a volcano of violence. Which is so easy to get dragged into. I had eleven hostages myself. Three of them were wing governors. A doctor. Even my own lawyer. The list goes on. Your Bob worked with the worst. But amazingly helped so many. Just how amazes me.

Anyway Sue, go for it. It's a sure winner. Also be a nice pension for you and Bob. Go on a world cruise. I don't believe there's another book like it. My respect to Bob.

January 2023
HM Prison Woodhill

The author of the Foreword

Charles Bronson (Aka Salvador) has spent decades in maximum security prisons and hospitals often in solitary confinement or segregation, including Parkhurst, Wormwood Scrubs, Wakefield, Gartree, Bellmarsh, Rampton, Broadmoor and Ashworth. Variously dubbed Britain's most 'dangerous', 'feared', 'notorious' and 'violent' prisoner his eclectic involvements include being a bare-knuckle boxer, minder, fitness fanatic, violent offender, hostage-taker, rooftop protester, award-winning artist, cartoonist, poet and author of around 20 books including *Loonology: In My Own Words* (2008). His life story formed the basis for the biopic *Bronson* starring Tom Hardy. Bronson 'befriended' Sue and Bob Johnson after 'Dr Bob' engaged with him to gain his 'painful trust' and respect as described in *Chapter 2* of this book.

Prologue

I was in that delicious state of relaxation when I knew that I was just dropping off to sleep. The telephone rang. Bob stirred beside me. Many years of doctor training and on-call nights served him well. Resisting all but the most imperative sound, he pulled the duvet closer, clutching at sleep. I picked up the phone.

'Sue speaking.'

'Is that Mrs Johnson?'

'Yes.'

'This is a C-Wing officer. I shouldn't be telling you this, but could you tell Dr Bob to watch his back?' a young male voice said urgently and quickly. 'H is threatening to kill him tomorrow.'

'Oh alright', I replied, an automatic response that was neither true nor real. It was anything but alright. The phone clicked off.

I nudged Bob. 'That was C-Wing. H is threatening to kill you tomorrow.'

Bob grunted... focused. 'Nothing to do now. I'll deal with it later.' He turned over and resumed his sleep.

My stomach twanged. My head hurt. I felt sick. *What was this?* I knew enough about the prison system by now to recognise that threats like that were dealt with swiftly. The prisoner was immediately sent to the Segregation Unit and brought before the Governor on a GOAD (Good Order and Discipline) charge. *What was going on? Why wasn't this happening? Why did the officer say he shouldn't be telling? Why ring now at 11.30 pm?* I supposed it was a change of shift to nights. *He was on his own. He could ring without his colleagues knowing. Bob's direct private emergency phone number was in the officers' station on the wing.*

I knew too that H was serious and well capable of slaughter. He'd killed staff in prison before, which was why he was on this experimental psychiatric wing of a maximum-security prison. It was also why my dear Bob was there, to treat him. I'd met H, shook his hand, and noticed the scars around his neck and across his arms, his clever but untouchable gaze. A spasm of uncharacteristic and fearful rage shook me. I wanted to march into the prison, grab him, shake him and say, 'What are you doing? Bob is only trying to help. Say sorry!' I remembered when our three children were small and being bullied by a larger boy on the way to school. I'd confronted him, saying he was being nasty and frightening. That bully had said sorry—but this… this was something I couldn't handle, something from which I couldn't protect Bob, and it hurt.

I left Bob sleeping and went downstairs. He would need his wits about him in the morning. I padded about the kitchen. *This is ridiculous, how the hell did I end up like this, with my husband on a serial killer's hit list, and me impotent to do anything?* Hot milk and grated nutmeg are said to be calming. I reached for the nutmeg and started grating. *Hell! I've grated my knuckles now.* Sucking the knuckle, I grumbled angrily. *Proper people have proper lives, with proper nutmeg graters, it's time I had a nice, elegant silver one.* A memory came glancing into my mind of Bob telling me that nutmeg trees were only growing in one place in the whole world until the 1850s, and that this was a clue Robert Louis Stephenson had given to the location of Treasure Island.

I wandered outside and looked across the dark garden to the leaden sea beyond, illuminated by a coldly clear moon: a hauntingly beautiful scene. I thought of H in his cell, and wondered when he had last seen the moon, and felt a sharp night breeze. I remembered my naïvety when I'd supposed that prisoners could at least see the stars from their cells and been told that the floodlights around the prison made it impossible. I wondered if H was as sleepless as I was, and if even now he was plotting my husband's murder. I knew that a characteristic of his was to plan, and plan…

Why didn't the prison seem to want to protect Bob? And how on earth did we two get here? And what will happen tomorrow?

CHAPTER 1

The Beginnings

Eighteen months earlier

I liked my office at Manchester Metropolitan University. Though small, it had room for four comfy blue chairs, where much conversation with colleagues took place. It was on the very top floor, and there were wide views from its large, functional if inelegant windows.

Gazing down over the busy cityscape I had felt a stirring sense of satisfaction. It was 9.30 on a Friday morning in March 1991. I'd sorted the day, battled the traffic and felt the usual relief that my early start had secured a parking spot, as well as control of the coming day. Walking past the slender, gently waving saplings on the path from the car park, I had recognised happiness. The joy of having a job where I could share ideas and innovate was still fresh. Struggling out of the glue of university politics, I had fashioned a small unit that operated on a wide scale. Supporting the one thousand academic staff of the university with personal and professional development opportunities and advice, it also ran European-funded courses for professional women returning to work, and organized teacher training courses for lecturers. My doctoral research into the philosophy and practice of education was also progressing.

At 49 I was 'still lively', two words that came to hold such meaningful resonance in the unforeseen struggles to come. Lively because I really did feel newly sprung, work until recently having been negotiated around the needs of my three children. I was just about to go for coffee and talks about my latest idea, 'Brokerages of Experience', when smashing into all my expectations the telephone rang. It was Bob, my husband of twenty-five years. Bob, the interesting, captivating, disrupting, challenging, maddening, and loving presence in my life.

When we met, I had just left university, and after a somewhat dismal time with a series of affairs that had more to do with sex than relationship, was convinced that marriage was oppression. A close friend at university almost died after an illegal abortion. This frighteningly shattering event pushed my growing and angry feeling that there was little place for a woman in the world, and an even lesser place for a married one. Back then, of course, we were called 'ladies' without irony, and denied mortgages and loans in our own names, let alone abortions and contraception.

But then I encountered Bob, a fledgling psychiatrist. His optimism, idealism, intellect and kind brown eyes engaged my trust, my understanding and then my love. This was someone with whom I'd never be bored, and what's more he was writing a book, *The Elusive Horizon*, and agreed with me that Wittgenstein was overblown. Tall, strong and handsome, he was nevertheless the opposite of macho man, and played Schubert with a haunting sensitivity. It spun circles in my youthful heart, magnified by the notions of equality, peace, and compassion we so shared.

And now his voice on the other end of the phone was saying, 'I think I might have to work here. Can you come down?'

'What?!!'

'It's just I think I could do it all here.'

My stomach lurched. 'Here' was Parkhurst, a maximum-security prison on the Isle of Wight. Bob had never been *in* a prison, let alone *worked in* one.

'Can you come down and see?' he continued urgently. 'It's Saturday tomorrow, and John says he will take you into Parkhurst and show you round.' John was the bouncy 'Number One', the Governor in supreme charge of the entire prison. Prisons have many governors; governors in charge of accommodation, governors in charge of security, of education, of building works, of wings, but the greatest of accolades is simply Number One, reserved for the person in powerful charge of the whole lot. John was the youngest Number One ever, a star in the Prison Service firmament, charming and not above a spot of managerial manipulation when occasion demanded. He was also the new partner of an old friend of mine. She and I had trained together years ago. I enjoyed her sparky, irreverent company, and Bob and I had recently stayed with them in their new home on the Isle of Wight.

I was remembering now a conversational challenge during that visit, between a dinner guest—*Lock 'em up and throw away the key. Born evil*—and Bob—*No, it's the long-term effects of child abuse, they can change.* Then John—*I am running the only Psychiatric Wing in the country. We manage people Broadmoor can't.* I had got the impression that this C-Wing Unit was a definite feather in a liberal careerist prison governor's cap.

So John subsequently invited Bob down to see how they ran the unit. Bob of course, always curious, went, but not before we had a conversation about how impossible it would be to work in a dungeon so this was a bit of a stunner. After over twenty-five years of life with Bob I knew his words and actions were never idle. *What was this leading to? I've just had the kitchen done for the first time, for god's sake, and I like the green marble tiles. My job is great. It suits me. It has been a hard-won trek.*

What do you wear in a maximum-security prison, and especially on a special unit for dangerous psychopaths? Prison officers wear uniforms, other staff suits, but what does the visiting psychiatrist's wife wear? I picked out a slightly swinging knee-length skirt, a white blouse, and the jacket which I had bought in America after my suitcase of clothes had been lost at the airport. *What else?* I fixed a silver leaping-deer brooch to the lapel, a present from my eldest daughter. *Was the deer gracefully leaping over obstacles or was it running for its life?*

Sitting in the early-evening train from Manchester to London on the first leg of my unexpected journey to the Isle of Wight, I speculated on John's motives. It was clear he was trying to get Bob to work there. But why was he bothering? Although fully qualified and a member of the Royal College of Psychiatrists, Bob was in no sense a standard consultant: he'd been blacklisted for refusing to give electric shock treatment, hence his leap into general practice, and his pursuit of the importance of family relationships and early trauma on emotional distress.

I just didn't know enough. I was tired and overwhelmed by the looming implications of what Bob might be proposing.

My first time inside a prison

Arriving at Portsmouth Harbour from Waterloo, I caught the Fast Cat to Ryde Pier Head. It had been a long day. I was so anticipating seeing my dearest daffy one, but it was John waiting there, no Bob, no urgent debriefing, no reassuring hug, what was up?

'Bob went to Cowes to meet you. Couldn't stop him, he got mixed-up—thought you'd be on the Red Jet', John said, with a grin just short of delight I thought.

Stopping for a bottle of wine on the way back to his farmhouse home John was all charm and laughs. 'It will be great having Bob around, we can make waves. It's important and unique work. The island is a great place to live. Houses are cheap. You will love it.' All I wanted was to see Bob and prepare to face the unknown reality of Parkhurst the next day.

Getting out of the car the next morning, Bob and I walked over to where John was waiting for us by the gatehouse. This part of the prison was new. The clean red bricks seemed to go upwards forever. Getting nearer I looked up. The walls were topped by a monstrous bulbous overhang which seemed to block out the sky. It was wound around with funny looking wire, quite thin, not the barbed wire I had expected. I later learned that this was called razor wire, capable of cutting anyone to pieces. In the distance I glimpsed a uniformed man with an Alsatian on a lead. As the man approached, John explained that there were regular patrols around the external perimeter, cheerily fed the dog a crisp, and pushed open the door to the waiting gatehouse.

John had briefed his staff well as I now know, and unusually we didn't go through any security clearance, no patting down, no removal of belts, no endless waiting for steel doors to be opened. Even so it was a shock. Inside the gatehouse was a kind of airlock watched over by prison officers who quickly activated the first set of sliding gates. They clunked behind us as we entered the enclosure, briefly imprisoning us at the whim of the watching officers. The gates ahead slid open. John chatted affably to the officers, and picking up his key, waved a big tag marked 'Number One.' Then we were off into the bowels of the place, accompanied by respectful officers who kept our passage smooth. Designed to be frightening, it *was* frightening.

After leaving the quickly unlocked door of the administrative block we were in the internal outside space of the prison, crisscrossed with hugely tall wire fences and heavy barred metal gates. Surprisingly there was a lovely little hedge in one of the compounds, sheltered by the wall of one of the old prison blocks. John stopped for a chat with a solitary prisoner who was gently and carefully trimming it. The hedge had little pink flowers, and was semi-hardy, but thrived in this climate, the man informed us. *What else would? Rabbits wouldn't stand a chance,* I thought, distracting myself momentarily from the nature of this walk to work. I wasn't to know then that the hedge didn't stand a chance either.

After three more unlocks, C-Wing was before us, and another airlock-type set of gates, and then we entered what felt like an underground tunnel: the Special Unit. *Is this going to be special for Bob, and in what way? The air isn't fresh. The light isn't natural. The smell is institutional. The sounds aren't soft.*

I hung back and looked around. A large, somewhat stout officer came directly over to me: 'Just look at that lot. You wouldn't think they were the most dangerous men in the whole prison system. Murderers, and more', he bragged casually. 'We call that the happy hatch. That's where they get their drugs.' I looked across to where there was a small hatch, and a line of about a dozen men slouching against the wall. They were different shapes, different heights, different ages, but the line itself exuded an air of sullen and absolute despair. *What brought them here?* I wondered.

The line looked at me with the faintest glimmer of interest. I raised my hand in acknowledgement. So that was it. Bob was to be the prescription pen for the dishing out of these drugs. I later learned that these men were consuming a truly record breaking 3.5 kilograms of drugs every year. *How could Bob's intense talking therapy possibly prevail?*

For those waiting at the happy hatch there were drugs for sleeping: chloral hydrate and Mogadon. Drugs for psychosis: stelazine, sulpiride, chlorpromazine, haloperidol and modecate. Drugs for anxiety: Valium and Librium. Drugs for depression: imipramine, amitriptyline. There were blue ones, yellow ones, white ones, multi-coloured ones. Some were tiny, some large, some had delayed action, some were immediate. They all had to be swallowed in front of the watching officer. Hence the queue. And of course, there was always the injection.

The chemicals flooding the men's minds were to be yet another unanticipated battle.

I moved on into the gloom and down the wing, following the important little gang that was surrounding Bob and John—the principal officer, T, always an ultra-correct respectful step behind John, the wing governor, the chief medical officer, the deputy wing governor, and the nosy dispensing officer untroubled by his waiting queue. Other ranks looked on. It was clear that Bob's visit the day before had made a big impression, quite what sort I didn't know, but they were assuming he was soon to join their merry band of hardy troops, and that my visit was purely placatory. I was not to be allowed to see the deeper horrors that Bob told me he had been introduced to. The men who were held in extra special conditions, dubbed 'The Real-life Hannibal Lecter' and other terrifying names. *Therapy in these conditions, I think not—oxymoronic or what? More like moronic to even try.*

We trundled on past a recreation area, complete with padded leatherette bench seats, foam poking out of the odd rip, and irony of ironies, a fish tank for a surprisingly small piranha. The stairs to the 'Ones', as the cells on the first floor were called, loomed upwards out of the middle of the wing. A classic sight for anyone used to prison dramas. Metal and ugly, they were draped from landing to landing with black suicide netting, spread out to break the fall of desperate men hurling themselves from the landings above.

Suddenly there was a clattering sound and a young man in a bright blue jumper appeared at the top of the stairs with a swiftness of purpose at odds with the surrounding doleful lethargy of the other prisoners. He ran down the stairs, crossed in front of the Governor, who equally ignored him, and walked briskly up to me.

Taking off his sunglasses he said, 'Will you let him come?' To this day I wonder what other direction our life would have taken if I hadn't been asked this. The appeal, the connection, the meaning were impossible for me to ignore. He had the air of a manager confident in his domain and his purpose. Looking at him, I nodded slightly. Satisfied, he turned away and went back up the stairs. I wasn't sure if anyone else except Bob even noticed. *What was it he noticed that made him pick out with such surety what he needed to do?*

Tour over, we headed back to the admin block. Getting out seemed somehow more oppressive than getting in. Reaching the air lock at the entrance to the wing we acknowledged the officers in their insulated glass-enclosed surveillance kiosk, from where they could keep the whole length of the wing, and the men, under observation. Once inside the admin block, normality asserted itself with ordinary clothes, open doors, women at desks, but the killer difference was the absence of what I realised was a pervasive wire-coiled tension—a tension that could snap at any time, not reducible by any amount of cheerful bonhomie.

The Beginnings

John ushered us into his office and took his place behind the most enormous desk I had ever seen. Swinging gently in his seat he pointed to a model of the prison that squatted on gleaming mahogany in a corner of the desk. It was complete with miniature Alsatians. *Miniature prisoners were probably too much reality,* I thought fleetingly. Picking up one of the dogs John was cheerfully expansive.

'Well, what do you think of the place?' Then, repositioning the dog, he waved his secretary in with the coffee.

Coming out, the prison behind us, I gulped in the early summer air. Kinder and softer than up North, it promised delights to come. *Out of sight, out of mind* came into my head. *Was that ever really possible? What would it actually be like for Bob, walking into that place every day?* I looked at him, certainly not out of his mind, or mine, though our friends were to tell us we both definitely were.

We were staying with John that night before going back to Manchester the next day, but first we had to talk and think, so we drove down to Cowes seafront. Parking on the esplanade, we slipped a pound into the parking meter and walked over to the elegant blue railings separating us from the sea below. I looked at Bob. He seemed full of a repressed eagerness, like a racehorse in the starting gate readying for the off, its training done, its goal the rich seam of misery, trauma and distress waiting to be defeated. 'I think I could work there', he said, and tentatively, 'What do you think?'

I leaned on the railings and gazed out at the sea. It was a busy seascape. As I watched the Red Jet Passenger Ferry sped past, followed shortly afterwards by the looming bulk of the car ferry, passengers waving from the open deck. The pale face of a ten-year-old boy crept into my mind. *He had the same look I had seen that day, the abandoned despair of needing help that never came.* The boy was in a locked ward of an American State Hospital having killed both his parents. I was teaching him to read.

'If you are right, it will work there, and if it works in Parkhurst, it will work anywhere', I said, remembering too that other locked ward in New York City, housing corridors of cages, the men inside calling out to me.

Over twenty-five years ago now, eager to embrace the future and each other, we had married in a gentle Quaker meeting house. Shortly afterwards, clutching visas and the green cards allowing us to work, we departed for the United States of America, at that time seen as an exciting, welcoming country at the cutting edge of psychiatric practice. The world was our gleaming oyster. I would teach, graduates from England were excessively valued then. This brief but powerful time together was to last two years before we came home to continue our careers and raise our family.

Bob had only recently returned from a States-wide study tour with a greatly strengthened view of the importance of his therapeutic discoveries, and was seeking a place to teach, research, test and develop his approach. Never could I have imagined it was to be in a dungeon! Some sort of community day centre was in my reckoning. Standing there on that holiday isle, surrounded by cheerful leisure seekers, we hugged each other very tightly, thinking of the future and, it seemed to me, the almost surreal challenges ahead. We could anticipate some. The danger of even attempting to explore the inner details of these dangerous men's minds, the sceptical antagonisms of the uniformed officers, the remorseless bureaucracy. Bob was anything but a company man, and here was the most archetypal company of all, hierarchical and rule-bound to its very core. *How could he — how would he — possibly survive?*

These, however, were to be the least of the perils…

A dinner party

That evening over dinner it was all hilarity. John and my sparky friend were lovely hosts. We ate asparagus from the garden, and some of the frozen glut from last year's delicious raspberries. Bob was in the trap and couldn't wait to get started. John had landed the fish he needed. They were both relieved and happy. As the newly arrived Number One Governor for this most flagship of prisons, John had succeeded in his boast of getting a psychiatrist for C-Wing, a position vacant for four months prior to his arrival. I could well believe it. A position not in the NHS, so no career there! And requiring residence near the prison. Additionally, 'It isn't a full-time post at this moment', John said vaguely, 'but we can sort all that out when you've got started.' A contract never did materialise. I wasn't to know, however, just how fortuitous this omission would turn out to be.

As the conversation progressed, I began to learn the importance of C-Wing. There were a few other Special Control Units, but this was the only one that was set up to deal with serious psychiatric conditions. It was envisioned as a solution to the 'mad axe-man problem.' These were the people who, though clearly mad, were labelled 'not mentally ill' by the psychiatric profession, and they were therefore considered untreatable and incurable. The Control Review Committee, set up by the Prison Service to advise on how to avoid riots, identified these people as triggers for prison disturbances. The recent Strangeways Prison riots in April 1990, and the ensuing report by Lord Justice Woolf, had refocused attention on this strategic role. I remembered the disturbances well, the rooftop protests, the deaths, the injuries. The causes were the subject of much safe arcane debate around the university coffee cups, but this was no such safe debate: somehow, I had slipped out of the calm of academia into a real-life drama.

'The Special Unit', John stated confidently, 'is a safety valve for the whole of the prison system, we manage the most dangerous violent and destructive of the lot.' I realised it was not just a Parkhurst resource, but a national one, with its own Special Unit Selection Committee (SUSC), meeting in London. It sifted requests from other prisons and selected the worst for incarceration in C-Wing. A psychiatrist was deemed essential to this plan, and since the beginning there had been constant difficulties in attracting such a person. John had indeed secured some brownie points.

Driving home the next day, we talked of practicalities. How was this going to work? Do I come to you at weekends? Do you come to me? Where do we live? John and his partner had offered Bob lodgings until it was sorted. Bob was his usual adamant self. 'We need a house. I will need to be on my own. I need to eat my own bread and porridge in the morning, and to grow bean sprouts.'

I really understood what he was saying. The intensity of the work he was about to embark on meant he needed to be able to totally relax without any worries about small talk niceties. Living with John would be living on the job, however well they got on. And it was true they were enjoying each other's company: they both had Tigger-like qualities of bouncing optimism, and for the moment John was relishing displaying what he called 'the social work and counselling side' of his job.

We fixed on the first of July for Bob to start, two months hence. This coincided with the start of my long summer break. The Isle of Wight had twice the sun, and half the rainfall of our northern home, and I was anticipating a summer of sunny relaxation, as well as, of course, encouraging chats with Bob about his job that I couldn't deny was, after all, really interesting.

We needed a house for Bob, and John pushing and pushing, needing to somehow contract me into the deal, astonishingly found the perfect place. The opposite of the dark northern millstone grit of our family home, this was a light early Victorian holiday villa, overlooking the sea. Its gardens hosted plants I could never grow up North, magnolia, arbutus and passion flowers. The sea's restless waves soothed my listening ears. It was indeed lovely, a place for holidays and a haven for Bob. I noted the cheerful certainty John gave his persuasive powers. He never doubted that our decisions were all down to his remarkable ability. John's new partner was my friend, a stylish urban sophisticate, an independent career woman who had given up her job to move to the island with John: I'm sure he thought I would be good company for her, and incidentally justify his persuasive tactics. What wasn't there to like?

So, granted a second mortgage on the basis of my salary, we rather miraculously bought and took possession of our new home just two months later at the start of my long summer break. The weather was glorious, and naïvely I was looking forward to a holiday.

The first week

It was the beginning of many a battle-chat with Bob, starting with the suit question. He had to have one, 'simple but not easy', as he would say of his therapy: Bob was tall, very tall, and hated wearing suits. He hadn't even worn one at our wedding. However, he was surprisingly resolute about this. 'It's a question of respect for the men', he said, 'I need to show them I'm a serious man, doing serious work with them. I am not a liberal do-gooder, trying to show I am on their side by wearing a jumper.'

This was to be his first move towards the trust he knew he needed. Grey wouldn't do, John always wore a grey suit. Pinstripes, that's for the lawyers, not shiny, that's the city trader, wide guy. Luckily, High and Mighty, the only shop that had suits that could even remotely fit him, had a plain dark navy one. It was this suit that was to define my image of him as he entered the prison on that first day, a man who knew what he was about.

His first task was to interview the men, take histories and assess the size of the problems. To his astonishment there was no office for him. *What? All that fuss, all that manoeuvring,.. all that energy to get him here, and no office! This was supposed to be an experimental psychiatric wing, the only one in the country.*

'There's never been a need really', said the wing governor. 'The previous psychiatrist used to sit in the dispensary over there behind the happy hatch. He loved playing his guitar, and the men seemed to like it too.' Then dismissively: 'But you can use the probation officer's room I suppose.' *Of course he could!* The probation officer rarely used it. There was no need there either, the men were going nowhere. Not for them any real sentence plan. Directionless, they had come to a full stop.

'I'll get their files and round them up', he continued, bristling with command. 'You'll probably get through them all in a day. They'll never come, of course, they'll have to be ordered.' Assertive, with a brisk confidence, he was an upright, handsome man, unnaturally tanned, of middling years with an athlete's physique. None too bright, he was scrupulously role precise. John called him 'Mogadon', after the sleeping pill of the day, a type of hilarious cruelty which seemed to me to be the off-duty default mode for those working within the prison system.

Bob was firm. 'Actually no. Ask them whether they want to see me. And I'd like everyone to call me Bob. And I don't want to see the files, just the prescription records thanks.'

'As to the prescription records, you'll have to see the dispensing officer about those.' Bob was startled to find that how he wished to be named was viewed with absolute, adamant and grim refusal, bordering on aggression by all the uniformed staff. It just could not be allowed. It implied disrespect, lack of control, lack of everything they took a pride in. Bob compromised. 'Call me Dr Bob.'

The next dispensing officer objected. Dispensing was his domain. He'd had special training after all, and no-one else had ever needed to see *his* records. I recalled his shape, and his demeanour: stocky, aggressive, a well-judged fraction short of rude. I sighed, but Bob was determinedly clear, 'I got them in the end. He couldn't absolutely refuse. I am their doctor, after all.' Suddenly and sadly, I could picture the conflicts to come that this foretold. *They don't deserve a doctor. Bob shouldn't be giving the scum a professional review of their treatment.*

The drugs are for control, pure and simple — what does that idiot psychiatrist think he's meddling with?

Thus the challenges of those first few weeks were laid down, exposed by this seemingly simple interchange. The men *were* their files. They were absolutely defined by what was written about them in page after page, year after year, of formulaic observations, something akin to structured gossip. Voyeuristic and toxic, they provided no clues for Bob's quest, but to ignore these files was seemingly to ignore the labour, the work of countless psychologists, probation officers, personal officers, wing governors: the file is what they *did*. These multitudes of staff used them to construct further records to go in the files. Through the files accountability could always be placed for any horrific events that were always lurking around. The files were evidence for whatever narrative was needed, a pick-and-mix smorgasbord of chilling treats. Throughout Bob's career within the prison and the courts these files were a constant source of antagonistic debate.

Bob knew the men's histories were horrific, far beyond any comfortable imaginings, but the details he was after were about the current workings of their minds; trust and consent were the essential stepping-stones for him in this most coercive and controlled of environments. In any event Bob persevered and went round making appointments. Some men refused, but most did not, whether out of curiosity, boredom, the chance to create some problems, or to access some form of help, it was too soon to know.

An office was rather more problematic and Bob appealed to John, who decreed that Mogadon's office be returned to its original two-cell condition, authorising prison works to build a brick wall down the centre. This must have been bruising for Mogadon, as he subsequently requested a transfer and moved off the wing. Nevertheless, the building works took months, and only commenced after repeated formal reminders from Bob to John. The electrics never were sorted, and the lights in Bob's office remained under the control of the adjoining half of the former office.

All the offices on C-Wing were formerly cells, and so had identical configurations. The probation office was no exception. It had a small window, with bars, through which Bob had to push his hand if he wished to open it, but also, chillingly, a deep sloping window ledge built into the inside wall to make suicide attempts by hanging from the bars more difficult. It was here I pictured Bob starting his venture, sitting with his back to the wall, the shape of its brick construction only just showing after decades and decades of layers of glossy cream paint. Parkhurst was a very old prison, built to house children about to be deported. Most of the doors were unusually short, and Bob had to stoop more often than usual.

At the end of that first week a drama occurred which could well have ended this story right here.

CHAPTER 2

The Strong Man

I knew about Bronson. John had jovially regaled us with gruesome, and not-so-gruesome tales of this man's exploits during that momentous supper party a scant few months ago, when we were staying with him for what we had blithely assumed to be a bit of a holiday. At that time, I learnt Bronson had been in prison for all but a few weeks of his adult life, and most of that in isolation within segregation units. It seems he was considered one of the most dangerous men in the prison system, and John's Parkhurst was the top of the tree on that score. The place that was big enough to manage these men. He was excited, and proud to be governing the prison that could house them. I had observed his delight in obtaining these volatile men. They provided a total justification for all that extensive security and immense expense, a compelling reason for much of the macho training. John himself was one of the trained national hostage negotiators, ready at any time to gallop off to what was termed an 'incident' at any prison in the country. He had shown us some sort of small black box, kept ready for when he received the summons.

It was an unusual and interesting dinner party conversation. I could see Bob thinking and wondered whether he'd disclose his thoughts or let the banter continue. It was all irritating me a bit. I looked at him. 'What would you do? Could you treat these men?' Bob was serious, really serious. 'Yes', he said. The reaction around the table was not even sceptical. I could see them thinking *Bob's just being silly, he can't possibly mean it, it's just an extreme debating point.* They were wrong of course. Bob never used words idly, and expected others to know that. I knew this characteristic from my very early days with him. John sensed this and had pushed the challenge: 'Some of the prisoners I have to manage have killed in prison, what's the point of prison for them?' For the most part the dinner table was incensed: 'What!! Prisons can't stop prisoners killing. They should lock them in solitary for life. It's a pity there's no death penalty.' And I had murmured mildly: 'It does rather show the failure of a "prison works" policy. Didn't a previous Home Secretary say, "Prison is an expensive way of making a bad situation worse?"' Then John, looking at Bob: 'We must always treat prisoners with humanity.' 'Yes', said Bob, nodding. 'They can change, and I know the roots of their violence lie in how they have been treated.' John laughed ... rather too loudly, I thought, and the table, relieved, followed his amused dismissal of a too-serious challenge.

When Bob started work that first week, I was somewhat relieved to think he wouldn't yet be facing the worst of the worst that this dinner party chatter had painted. Those men were segregated, locked away in their own particular dungeons. Instead, I pictured him on C-Wing. The men I had seen there, though undoubtedly dangerously, violently volatile, were also vaguely familiar, a bit like sullen institutionalised, suspicious psychiatric patients on locked wards. *Besides they were being constantly monitored by officers who would surely spot trouble and tell Bob*, I reassured myself.

However, Bob had been in the prison for only four days when I heard the clanging metal of our garden gate. It was stiff and noisy after Bob had fixed an extra strong spring to keep out the badger who had been messily scavenging our dustbins. So, a bit of an early warning system then. I tried to quieten the sudden lurch in my stomach and looked at Bob anxiously as he came through the kitchen door. This wasn't normal, he looked a bit grim. *Where was the cheerful smile, the hug, our usual exchange of pleasantries—How are you doing? What's going on? How have you been today?—followed by 'Fine', and anecdotal exchanges*. No. This was different, very different.

Bob switched on the plastic lime green kettle. I had bought it for a bit of fun, ideal for a holiday home by the sea. Our sensible heavy duty black one was of course still in our Manchester home.

'I saw Bronson today. It didn't go well.' Bob was thinking and thinking. 'I'm not sure what it was ...'

'What?' I cut in, wilfully interrupting his thoughts. 'What the fucking hell are you on about? Bronson isn't in C-Wing. You're not supposed to be seeing him yet, you've only been in the prison five fucking minutes! Bronson kidnaps for fun, for interest, to fill his time, you don't know any of their daft rules, you don't know Bronson for God's sake. Where did you see him? Were the officers with you?' I was ranting and scared.

Bob was firmly unshaken. 'It's alright... I'm alright... it's going to be alright, don't worry.'

'What do you mean it didn't go well? What did Bronson do?'

Bob seemed somewhat cross with himself and was puzzling to understand what had gone wrong. 'He tore up the notes I made on him.' And with relief: 'Not the ones of all the others...'

I knew how precious these notes were for Bob. He'd been carefully interviewing the men all week, and they contained his vital first thoughts. He had gone down to the Segregation Unit as John had asked him to interview Bronson. The debate was now real. The college boy was being tested. The dinner party seminar was to be played out in a living context. Would safety reside in human and informed relationship, or burly manpower?

Bronson was in isolation, continually watched. His latest infraction against GOAD was to tear down the central heating pipes, and to charge down the corridor with a wing governor stuffed under his arm. He was unnaturally strong. Bob described him as looking a bit like Captain Webb, the nineteenth-century cross-channel swimmer. He had turned his body into a destructive threat through hour-after-hour, year-after-year of relentless press-ups in his lonely cell. Staff and prisoners rightly respected this threat.

Officers had escorted Bronson from his cell to the interview room and stationed themselves at the door. Bob and Bronson were seated on opposite sides of a long narrow table that ran down the middle of this converted cell, at right angles to the door. There was no panic button, I discovered.

'We officers are there. Just signal, and we'll be all over him.'

Well, they weren't. When Bronson stood up, and loomed over Bob, there was no-one to signal to. The officers had evaporated. Bronson grabbed the whole bundle of precious notes. 'Are these my notes?' he demanded. Bob appealed, 'Just the top two pages are yours, Charlie.' Pealing-off the top two pages, Charlie carefully, deliberately shredded them into one-inch squares before stalking out. The interview was over.

This must have taken some time. The A4 sheets were carefully torn into one-inch-long strips, then folded, torn, and refolded. I tried this at home. It took time. Each sheet produced a thick pile, and as I progressed I needed to separate the piles in order to shred them. However, I suppose Bronson, being so strong, would have been quicker, but the noise of the tearing paper was unmistakable.

A signal that should have been acted on. Bob told me he was about to pick up the shredded bits of paper, thinking he might be able to Sellotape them together, when an officer appeared. 'You won't be needing these then', he said with a smirk, and swept them up into the bin.

Shock and anger

I was shocked and angry. *What was this? Surely this couldn't be a spiteful and dangerous set up? What had stopped Charlie from murdering Bob?* Scared, a picture of a huge muscular man grabbing Bob by the throat and hurling him across the room hit my mind. I later learnt that this was more than a nervous wife's fantasies, it was a real possibility. Bronson documents in brutal detail his trail of violence and hostage-taking in his book. I learnt from this that he had attacked officers, trashed a wing, and got onto the roof of Parkhurst. John had spent hours talking him down, an action that Bronson had evidently respected.

Even some of the men on C-Wing were scared and had asked for his removal to the Segregation Unit. I couldn't believe John's folly. What had he been trying to prove? That Bob needed his protection? That his prisoners were evil and frightening? That he was the one that could control these men? That Bob would flee? I felt sick with fury and disbelief that John could be so frivolously reckless, and raged impotently at Bob, angrily scared. He was putting his theories before his life. 'What's the matter with you? Can't you see Bronson really could have throttled you?'

This first encounter with Bronson had lasted fifty-five minutes, and despite the frightening show, Bob was undismayed, and, I found out, undeterred, but I began to feel helplessly battered. This was all starting to demand a very new and unknown level of communication, of understanding, of support between us. *Were we — could we even be — would we be — up to it? And as for the rest: how would this type of lurking hostility play out, and could I really find a way of managing my sickening feelings?* I knew there would be lots more to come. I looked at this tall man sipping green tea from a large mug. Domestic details often eluded him, but he was unusually particular about his tea — just three or four leaves and no milk, an easy enough drink. But this wasn't going to be an easy enough conversation.

'What do you think about things?' I shouted fiercely, loud and cross.

I felt ill, feeble, wobbly. Pictures of what could've happened kept hitting me, and I couldn't rid myself of the notion that John was having a cruel joke. *Here was the Number One Governor of the most dangerous prison in the country, manager of a budget of millions of pounds, in supreme command of what amounted to a small, totally self-contained town, with its own security, its own kitchens, its own training, its own laundry, its own gym, its own chapel, its own education, its own administration, even its own operating theatre, sending someone who was completely inexperienced in prison protocol and rules, let alone its culture, into a confrontation situation with what he, and everyone else knew, was the most unpredictable and violent man under his command.* Bob looked at me. 'I think I'll just play the piano for a bit', he said.

He nearly always played Schubert. It suited him. It had layers of meaning. He was continually delighted at the variety of chords, and the difficulty. It was new every time, he would say. It was enticingly paradoxical music. I could hear it from my retreat in the darkening garden. Did I believe in this project? I imagined Schubert's belief, and his focus, such dedicated focusing and focusing on his music. He was never to hear his own symphonies played. I went back inside and hugged Bob.

'Who wants life to be easy? I didn't marry you to be bored.' He laughed, relieved. 'Oh thank goodness, open a bottle and we'll have a good chat. And', he went on, 'only three of the men refused to see me, even little C. So that's a good start. But I need a decent chair…'

Bob's increasing certainty

Amazingly, the fiasco with Bronson only served to confirm Bob's certainty. If he could work with Bronson, he could work with anyone, and he had seen the beginnings. 'It's like this', he mused, 'actually trusting me was painful… he knew he might… and somehow couldn't bear it… he's been moved, and moved… the "roundabout" they call it… he glimpsed a new vision… too hard to think of it… I was offering him a choice… he's never experienced this… but he was careful not to totally destroy it.'

I understood. Bronson was being offered a glorious lollipop he daren't grasp in case it was snatched away. Bob's urgent enthusiasm began to infect me. I glimpsed some of the vision. He was a doctor through and through, a clinician forged in a bygone age of enquiry. He was on a quest to find the cause and cure of dangerousness. He had chosen an area populated by condemnation and devoid of enquiry. Like the explorers of old, it was exciting virgin territory for him.

While Bob ordered for next-day delivery what I later came to think of as an iconic chair, my bit of bravado lurched up and down. I was still shaky. Not being bored was one thing, but total body-gripping scared nausea was quite another. And this fear I wasn't going to be able to defeat through my own action. It wasn't my ball to play. *Hell! I couldn't even be on the touchline. How to generate the strength? Did I even want to? Was it really my project? It's all too much. The energy and passion needed, could I find it? Did I even want to? My too-distant a role, discussing tactics, pointing out pitfalls, encouraging, understanding, was just too difficult. I have nothing to guide me, only my fears. I was not a natural bystander. For goodness sake, I was the granddaughter of a Quaker suffragette!* These black spaghetti tangles of thoughts were becoming dark, too angry. I wandered outside again, glass in hand. The moon gleamed through the trees. How can all this loveliness exist alongside the weeping horror that was Parkhurst, a few short miles away?

Can I do this? Could I be as certain as Bob? I really needed to know what he was experiencing. In short, I needed to see the men, and C-Wing, again. I tried to explain it to Bob. 'I need to see the whites of their eyes.' *But how?*

CHAPTER 3

Early Days

As we moved into the second week of my still anxious turmoil, I began to understand just how much Bob needed my presence, my understanding, my comfort, as he eagerly talked and talked, describing his thoughts, his day. The chair still hadn't arrived. The local phrase 'This is the island, after all' I began to understand, too. So, Bob was sitting on an armless plastic chair to conduct that devastatingly important first conversation with E. As Bob talked with me, I pictured him: far too tall for a basic chair, legs crossed, one large foot dangling. Then, pen poised, leaning forward with an intense concentrated listening, scribbling, questioning, as he met E for the first time. The big man looks at him sceptically, arms crossed. He's dressed in running shorts and grey-white t-shirt and trainers. 'It's hot in there', Bob explains.

E is huge, running to fat, with a large shaven head. He grunts noncommittally. Later E was to say, 'I thought you was a quack.'

Bob persists gently, 'What's your number one problem?' and then, probing, 'Have you got any fear and anger from childhood?'

E shifts uncomfortably: 'Don't take me off me injections. I need to keep on with me injections. I tried coming off them in February and the temper came back something dreadful.'

Then suddenly the big man stands up and waves his arms about. Bob is scared. E was between him and the door. 'I hadn't learnt to read violence then. I think it took me about six months.' E was actually only recalling an incident where he lost his temper.

In these early days Bob had lunch with John in his office. John liked to swap counselling stories and check on how the new boy was getting on. Quite how this activity was perceived in this most hierarchical of institutions, Bob was ridiculously unaware, I realised with a burst of affection. To him it was just a friend having lunch with a friend, but the effect of this on the tangled grapevine of the prison helped Bob, as no doubt John knew. He was to withdraw this privilege as his irritation with Bob's overarching focus grew. Being liberal was one thing, but John had to be the top liberal. He wanted Bob to show it, to see how crucial, important and difficult his job as Number One Governor was, and to commend him for it, to acknowledge his power and achievements.

The protective effect of John's friendship lasted throughout the first crucial weeks of that strange summer. The officers were choosing to humour Bob in his idiosyncratic wish to talk to the men. It was clear they were waiting for him to get fed up and for this silly experiment to come to an end. He now had his own keys, a signal of belonging to this happy band of incarcerators. 'So you are good for something', growled one, as Bob courteously held open a sliding gate to one of the air locks. Reporting this, Bob was determined and excited. 'The whole point is that their work will be easier, less dangerous, less stressful. It's like Beirut in there at the moment, you never know when something is going to kick off, but I am having some great sessions with the Baron. We'll see where that goes.'

I learnt that 'The Baron' was the young man in the blue jumper. He was the most respected man on the wing. Nothing escaped him, as I had found on my first visit. I began to understand his peculiar status: more like a manager than a gangster—more like a CEO than a mafia chief.

I was worried, a doom-laden worry I couldn't quite pull into focus. Everything was ludicrous, surreal, stupid. *What was Bob doing, walking into a mini-Beirut every day, thinking he could change things before they kicked off? Was he just floating in a bubble of his own conviction that was doomed to burst?* His extreme vulnerability had me by the throat. *Where was his support? Where were his allies?* Bob badly needed goodwill.

We meet the CMO

The chief medical officer, in charge of the Hospital Wing, as it was euphemistically called, was head medic for the whole prison including C-Wing. He was in the Territorial Army, and, it was rumoured, of the SAS branch. I could well believe it. He looked military, not medical. Relishing a fight, his hospital was where those believed to be off the scale of dangerousness were kept in cages in solitary confinement, and the CMO was the man to handle them. Many a prisoner had reason to fear him. Bob and he struck up an unlikely friendship. The CMO was interested in psychopaths — *Not surprising, the SAS must be stuffed with them,* I thought, somewhat sarcastically — but anyway, no matter, so was Bob! They were to talk over morning coffee about the origins of psychopathic behaviour, Bob describing, pronouncing on his ideas about frozen terror being at the root of destructive behaviour. The CMO, sceptical but admiring of Bob's fearlessness in talking to these men, uncovering their terrors, and attempting a solution.

One day, wanting to challenge Bob's fearlessness and belief, the CMO invited us both to his home. He wanted to show us a video of the first time CS gas was used to end a brutal hostage situation inside a prison, the prison he had previously worked in as the medical officer in charge. I later experienced the peculiar nature of this prison, and understood some of the tragic triggers of what I was about to witness.

I recognised the man in the blue jumper and felt myself retreating into a clenching stillness. I looked at the CMO's face, watching Bob, as the nasty, cruel drama unfolded on this all too grimy, grainy video. I wasn't sure what he was hoping for. *Was it for Bob to start to really hate the men he was working with? Did he want him to feel frightened when confronted with the living reality of such viciousness? Certainly, it was a gruesome test, but did he really want Bob to pass this unique exam? And what was my role? He knew Bob was determined and strong, so maybe I was there to transmit my horror and fear to Bob as the proverbial Achilles heel, the frail woman. So — he was looking at me as well!* But — a bit of a sneaky thought — *John had thrown Bronson at Bob, and well he, the CMO, could do one better. Was that it too? Ludicrous competition among the boys?*

The room was oppressive, stuffy, and lacking in any sort of charm. I really didn't want to be there, in this too-ordinary home, with its fitted carpet, coffee table and three-piece-suite, but I couldn't ignore what was happening on the silent screen in front of me, and the cold, almost gleeful description with which the CMO was torturing my ears. *Just in case I didn't get it. Didn't get it, for gods sake!* An angry, determined pity crept into me. *So, this was what it was all about. This bloody well never had to happen again, to anyone, anywhere!* It was a test all right, but I think I learnt a very different lesson from that expected.

The initiation over, Bob continued with those most unlikely of coffee morning seminars, for he had in his sights a shadowy figure in one of the hospital cages. A few other allies popped up. The prison chaplain always admired what Bob was trying to do and told him comfortingly that Bronson had said he would never have hit the doctor. The carpentry instructor was always cheerful and gave Bob practical tips as to how to find his way about, but that was it really for my dearest daffy one, as he continued to learn how to overcome the roots of their cruelty from the only people who actually knew.

The first murder threat

The chair still hadn't come, something about needing a new customer reference number as we were on the Isle of Wight not in Manchester; and there was no sign of Bob's office being created any day soon, but as that strange summer progressed Bob was relishing his new discoveries.

The familiar clunk of the garden gate was a bit earlier than normal.

'C threatened to kill me.'

'But I thought you were getting on well with him.'

Bob sat down on one of our new garden chairs. He looked disturbed. I felt a painful constriction somewhere, and an incongruous snatch of song seemed to roll in with the early evening air: *Somewhere over the rainbow, way up high… Oh… if only I could let all this float off over the seas and faraway, but no, this won't just float away.* I sat down and I listened. Just before lunch an officer had politely informed Bob of the murderous nature of the threat, and then disappeared. Lunchtime was when changeover meetings occurred, the officers relaxed, and the men were locked in their cells. When Bob returned from lunch officers met him.

'You have to talk to C. He's in the wing office.' Mogadon was nowhere to be seen, preferring a more literary role as wing governor. His managerial style was displayed through memos. This meant there was little check on the officers' cruder instincts. I remembered Mogadon: *Correctly incorrect, and perfectly useless to Bob.* 'You'll never change C', an officer had pronounced contemptuously. 'I have known him for ten years. He was born evil.' Proving the point, C was seated opposite Bob, growling, spitting, and flailing his arms about. 'What do you want to say to the doctor?' smiled a plump female officer, sitting perilously close to the chaotic C. I heard the incredulity in Bob's voice. He had

Early Days

been nervous for the woman, baffled as he was by this gross change—C had been one of the first to begin conversations with him.

'I was scared, but I apologised, and I think he'll come back', Bob summed it up, undeterred. I suddenly felt terribly, terribly weary. Not another set up! *Would this collision of cultures be the end of Bob?* I imagined the officers sniffing around the closed door of his office: they were trained to regard privacy as dangerous, and confidentiality as conspiracy. Everything about these men, their prisoners, had to be known. Their job was to know everything, to document it, to provide a continuing narrative of unremitting evil: *How dreadful for them then if, behind closed doors, an alternative narrative was being constructed which gave the possibility of transformation and dignity to such scum.*

CHAPTER 4

A Tea Party

More than ever, I needed to see these men again. I needed to see C, E, the man in the blue jumper, to see that shadowy line, to see if they really were responding. I couldn't share Bob's optimism. *How can I return to work without knowing it is going to be alright?* Feeling trapped, I yelled, 'Okay, okay, so he'll come back, so he'll smash you, so he'll strangle you, so nobody will help. The officers will wind it up and wind it up and wind it up. There's only me, and I'm useless, and I'm not going to be here anyway!'

'Sue. Sue. Don't. Don't. We'll go in and see them. You can find out for yourself. There's going to be a tea party on the wing. John said they need socialising, and you can be there.' He hugged me tight.

A tea party! What absurdity was this? A tea party!! What sort of small talk is appropriate? Done anything interesting lately? Yes. Just slaughtered an officer or two. What line of work are you in? Murder actually, quite good at it. Got some great write-ups. My imagination became fantastical. I wondered what I'd think this time around.

Bob wore a short-sleeved summer shirt and cream trousers. I was always trying to trim his beard. Too much like Freud I'd say, but it was difficult to get him to stay still for long enough. So today was only half of a job. *That's fine. That's OK. That'll do.* I wore a white shirt, nearly stylish with a shaped collar and a calf-length ecru-coloured cotton skirt. We looked, I suppose, middle-class, middle-aged and respectable as we set off for the party.

This time Bob had his own keys, and there was no John smoothing our way quickly forwards, so we waited in the gatehouse 'airlock.' I had no idea what we were waiting for, and felt suddenly and threateningly trapped, as the total extent of scrutiny and control hit me. Then the doors slid open, a number of officers entered, and we moved out and onto the first lot of metal gates. The protocol of opening, waiting and locking of these numerous gates was evident, and could clearly be used for much insidious harassment. I now knew why it could take Bob as much as half-an-hour just to get out of the place. Much later, I was to wonder just how the escapers, who were to have such a devastating impact on so many lives, could possibly have managed it.

Pink flowers and a piranha fish

So we went deeper into this dungeon of a village. I had supposed that accompanying Bob with his own keys would make it feel easier, but no, we were locking ourselves in the further we progressed. There was something about our choice in all this that disturbed me, but I smiled at the officers we met on this peculiar journey. They seemed somewhat embarrassed, and I sensed they liked Bob, a strong character who cracked jokes. This must have conflicted badly with their distaste for what Bob was doing.

I noticed the pink flowers on the hedge were beginning to fade, and indeed the hedge was much larger than I remembered it, stretching around the side of the block. I didn't notice anyone working there. As we emerged from the C-Wing air lock, an officer was standing ready to greet and escort us to the party. 'It's in the carpentry workshop', he said, ushering us forward. On the way I paused by the fish tank. 'The piranha looks a bit bigger', I said conversationally to the officer. Yes, he replied proudly, 'The men feed it with guppies from the other wings.' I thought it best not to side with the poor sodding guppies, and although there was no hint of it then, the piranha wasn't to make it either.

'Come on', said Bob, 'I'll introduce you.' John was already there. I felt myself feeling thankful. He was glad-handing himself around the room, his mass of wavy greying hair bobbing as he energetically nodded and chuckled, attempting to normalise the situation. King Canute sprung to mind, but I had to admire John's chutzpah, and of course he was right, the men did need socialising. Bob had told me that most of them had never ever had a meal with others: throughout their disastrous childhoods they were feral grazers.

I'd made the mistake of reading some of the lurid True Crime literature. I instantly recognised the man who was approaching and swallowed down a moment of gruesome nerves. I shook his hand. It was limp, and a bit damp. I recognised how hard he was trying. With an effort of unfamiliar, correct formality, he offered me a cup of tea and engaged in the strangest of conversations.

A Tea Party

'I have this ma lady', he began. I nodded, thinking addressing me as 'my lady' a bit too much really, but I didn't know what the social rules were either. 'But', he went on, 'then help descended', and he stretched out wide his long thin arms. I realised he meant *malady* and was referring to Bob's arrival on the wing. I listened with a pang to this solitary being, carefully educating himself in his cell and now practising for the first time words he'd never heard spoken.

They used to hang us here…

Quite suddenly he moved over into a smaller section of the room, a kind of annex framed by a wide archway. I followed, holding my tea. He was tapping his foot on the floor. 'Do you know what was under here?' he said, staring at me with a curious expression which to this day still haunts me. 'It's the gallows. They used to hang us down there.' I looked down at the comfortless institutional floor and twitched a bit. 'Oh dear', I said limply, and relieved to move away from that spot accepted a bun from a small thin little man who approached purposefully, holding out a plate of brown-looking buns in white paper cases. *Cupcakes seems to be a bit of a craze*, I thought, *with their multi-hued glittery sprinkles and iced hearts. There are shops that sell nothing else.* These, however, were their plainer cousins. I couldn't tell whether they even had a currant or two in them. He told me they'd made them specially in their kitchen and, following his gesture, I saw an arrangement with a cooker, sink and kettle, sufficient for drinks, and the odd snack. Thanking him, I observed, with a shock, ligature marks around his neck, and deep scars on both arms. 'Like ploughed fields some of them', Bob told me later. As I moved around the room these signs of brutal, painful harm came to seem unnervingly normal.

One by one these strangest of tea-party hosts came to greet me. R, a huge man with a square head and enormous feet, whose appearance had once caused John to wonder aloud if there was anything in phrenology after all, said 'Hello.' I shook his hand. *What was I seeing? What was I looking for? What reassurance could I possibly get from this ghastly cast of characters?* The Baron was gliding around the room, almost proudly watching. 'Dr Bob is doing OK', he told me. There seemed to be glimmers of hope in the room, or was I imagining it? A tall, large man, who Bob later told me was E, came up to me with Bob.

'I thought he was a quack', he said grinning, 'but he's alright is Dr Bob.' And he turned to Bob saying, somewhat mischievously, I thought, 'If you had said call me Doctor Johnson I'd have had nowt to do with you', and I knew he meant it, for all the grins he was deadly serious. A small boyish man with long hair and a silly smirk shook my hand. 'This is C', said Bob. *C! The man who'd threatened to tear Bob limb from limb was seeking approval!* There was just one man circulating on the outskirts of all this, whose hand I never got to shake. I later learnt just how dangerous he could be.

The party over, we returned home. I was exhausted. 'Well, did you get to see the whites of their eyes?' Bob joked seriously. 'Yes! Yes! I did', I said irritably. 'What do you think then?'

'I think they are all feral, adult kids who never grew up. Peter Pans in Gruesome Land', I said angrily. The truth hurt and as I spoke I could see those tiny, tiny needy, oh so needy little kids, but in huge grown dangerous bodies, and knew I wanted to give them a chance with Bob. I knew too that I had been somewhat reassured this whole mad quest might just be possible. *Was I deluded? I finally didn't want to be.* Bob knew that too.

CHAPTER 5

Trust and Change

The chair had at last arrived. It was functional, covered in a supposedly hard-wearing brown tweed-like cloth with padded leatherette on the arms. It had a high back, adjustable seat, and moved on castors. Suitably ugly I thought, as we heaved it into the back of the car, beginning its journey into the prison. I pictured Bob's lengthy trek pushing the chair on its revolving castors into his still-borrowed office. A 'there to stay' signal. I hoped it wouldn't rain while he was moving it. I didn't think he could expect much help.

Later that evening we talked, sipping a glass of wine as the late summer darkness slid over us. 'Well, we can't have a holiday for at least eighteen months', Bob mused, 'they're much too unstable. I need to demonstrate absolute total reliability. And total consistency. To have any chance of getting their trust, let alone their consent to explore the terrors.'

'Oh for god's sake Bob, you can't have forgotten the wedding! We need to be up there for at least three or four days, I want to decorate the Meeting House with bunches of heather. I've got all the white ribbon.' Lovely arrangements were well in hand. Our second daughter was getting married in a tiny historic Quaker Meeting House, and there was to be feasting and dancing afterwards. I was instantly mourning the loss of time with Bob. The sharing of a lovely weekend of happiness was going to be cut short. He was a great dancer, and our daughter had selected some of our favourite nostalgia. 'Moon River' was one.

'I know', said Bob, feeling the sacrifice. 'I have to leave the next day, but I'll manage most of it, and have breakfast with everyone.'

'Well at least we can dance in the evening.' Sad, I tried not to be cross as well. I wouldn't be able to have a lovely gossipy chat with him after the wedding either, I'd be off to Manchester, and it would be a long two weeks before I could manage a weekend in our island home again. So I returned to my work in Manchester, awaiting the next developments, and wondering how we would manage the looming practical, let alone emotional, tugs.

Growing enthusiasm

As the Ryde ferry swung alongside the pier bringing me to my next weekend rendezvous, I saw with a touch of excitement Bob's tall waiting figure. He has a wonderful smile, he looked so happy to see me my heart started to hurt. This really was difficult being so über-flexible.

'John's coming for supper tomorrow, if it's still as warm as this, I thought we might go down for a swim.' It was an enticing vision. Late-September, and the sea was still warm, but we weren't there for the sunshine. A picture of the prison, and those men waiting in that line sliced into my vision. I squeezed Bob's knee as we drove slowly off the elegant pier, built to enhance Queen Victoria's transportation to her holiday home. 'How's E doing?' Bob grinned. I could see how pleased he was. 'He's really getting stuck in. It's astonishing.' 'Great, I really want to see it.'

Just the day before at my university desk in far-away Manchester, pushing through the induction demands of fifty new lecturers, I had struggled with the import of Bob's excited telephone chatter. E had agreed to be filmed! The big man was making progress! 'It's a breakthrough, it's groundbreaking, it's hugely significant, and E trusts it all enough to let it be shared! He's the first! The others will follow!'

A burst of tired anger had shaken me. *Oh for god's sake*, I thought, *it's not the only thing that matters, bloody Parkhurst and bloody prisoners!* but Bob had rushed on, so beautifully confident in my silent support, 'You must see it next weekend.' He was right of course, I was engaged with the endeavour, whether it was Bob, or the prisoners, I was wearily unaware.

Trying to settle myself for sleep back in our old home, with the wind rustling the now-too-tall sycamore outside our bedroom window, I found myself plunging back into that prison world of misery, and the ludicrous hope Bob was offering. *What was so compelling in all this?* I wanted to see, and hear, what E was really like. *Was he as convinced as Bob? What sort of permission had he given? How could I support all this without really knowing? Was it really possible to know anyway, and what did I want to know?* Theoretically, I knew all the difficulties of evaluating therapy—observer bias, 'inter-rater reliability' and so on and so on—but Bob didn't do theory, and this wasn't theory, it was immediate, challenging and dangerous practice, reliant on trust. Trust in so bloody much more than just his own approach and experience.

The first video-recording

He needed trust in me, the prisoners, the prison system, John. All my professional knowledge, *Will I manage to gain some form of resolution from all this brain and heart hurt by watching the video of E?* I needed clarity, some answers. So, I was nervously anxious as I settled down with Bob to watch this very first video. *What if I can't agree, can't see what Bob is so excitedly chatting about?* Most of our belongings still being up North, the house was fashionably sparse, and the discomfort of our wicker sofa, purchased for its economy and lack of weight, echoed the discomfort in my mind. It was second-hand, and I noticed irritably little nails sticking out. The prevailing wind from off the sea rattled the windows in an early-Autumn warning. I'd been told it had an uninterrupted run all the way across the Atlantic from Brazil. I wanted to feel safe and I squeezed Bob's hand. He gave me an eager smile, then turned on the video.

'Well now E how are you doing?' 'Not so bad… and yourself?' This was the banal interchange that ushered in the least banal of any conversation and Bob's first radical use of video in the prison. Looking at the screen I was hit with the desolation of this big man and felt a shiver of fear as the frozen blank of his face stared at Bob. The environment in the cell was bleak and utterly, loomingly, enclosed with heavy, unadorned walls lit with unforgiving light. It was a mesmerising spectacle. Bob had placed the camera on its tripod just behind his left shoulder. It was perhaps this unwavering one-angled shot that added to the frozen quality of the scene. It was a bizarre tableau as E, unnaturally still except for the movement in his eyes, started to respond to Bob's insistent questioning.

Suddenly, my liberal imaginings evaporated as the harsh truth flooded in. I was seeing an ugly cell in a maximum-security prison. The door was closed. There was no panic button. Bob, wanting the light, was seated near the window, and a brooding thug who had killed for no known reason was between him and the door. I was scared. *What was he doing?! It's not a kindly GP consultation, this, it's actually dangerous. This is reckless, stupid.*

But as I watched I began to see the connection to Bob that this large, slumped, almost-but-not-quite-defeated figure, was nearly daring to believe as Bob vigorously, animatedly and with total conviction set about pumping life, hope and self-belief into him. Imagining what E was gazing at, I saw Bob in that ugly office chair, the seat accommodating his long legs, raised to its highest. He would be wearing the navy suit I'd so toiled to find, a white shirt, bright bow tie, and one of the pairs of Clarks strong slip-on black leather shoes, size twelve, bought to stay the course. Slightly hunched, he'd be leaning forward with a fixed and eager intensity of purpose... and the soft brown eyes, their kindness, and understanding, unmistakable.

He was engaged in discovering, and dissolving, the terror that was still driving the big man. The enormity of what E was experiencing suddenly grabbed me. This was beyond all his reasonings and experience. *Could he — would he — recognise it?*

The big man flinched, shielding his eyes with one stuttering hand. I saw a little, terrorised boy, and instinctively wanting to protect him from the terrors, thought *Stop, stop it, it's okay, don't worry,* but staggeringly Bob didn't. Instead, he was seeing the man, not the child. The man who, with support and understanding, could free himself from his terrors and begin to blossom, and it was the man who was starting to respond.

Later on I recall Bob sometimes referred to it as 'Blossom Therapy', a gentle, and hopeful title for a process that required so much courage, trust and penetrating enquiry, but — and it felt a fearsome 'but' — did E have the capacity to really trust that he could rid himself of the fear that had always governed his life at home, in care, in borstals and in prisons? Above all, did he really want to? As I looked at this burly prisoner, I was scared as well as interested. This was not a fiction being played on my screen. E could so easily hurt Bob. *What if he said the wrong thing, and pushed him too far?* But I thought too that somehow *he* was beginning to glimpse a choice and, ridiculously, I felt as though I was urging on a racehorse! *Go E, go!*

It was gripping. A powerful, and strangely illuminating conversation, neither interrogation nor kindly counselling.

Bob asks, 'How are you going to stop the fear?' And E, grasping for understanding, for relief, replies, 'I'm going to tell her... I am...'

'What are you going to tell her?'

'That I'm an adult.'

Suddenly the big man's voice seems clearer. He is gaining strength through saying the words, and follows this up with, 'Start talking nice, and all that. No shouting, like you normally do.' Bob, pushing on, says, 'Can you see that the anger went down when you understood where it came from?' 'Yes... you're brainwashed into fear.'

Bob's hand came into view. I noticed his wedding ring on long, strong, shapely fingers. E stood, grasped the hand, and turned to leave. He was wearing what seemed like running shorts. The film stopped, and a smiling face came into view, recording the time and date of the encounter. It had lasted eleven minutes. I didn't know whether it was a dream or a nightmare I'd been looking at. *Bob's dream, my nightmare perhaps.*

'So what do you think, you can see him changing, can't you?' said an eager Bob, secure in his own knowledge and experience, and anticipating my praise. Perversely I felt sudden irritation. *Me! Me! Where am I in all this?* I needed to trust myself, my judgement, and it wasn't clear. Questions and more questions tumbled around my assaulted brain. 'What do I think, what do I think?' I exploded, 'Oh, just get me some coffee.' Bob looked wounded, deflated. I was instantly sorry. It was courageous, inspiring, groundbreaking work he had just shown me, and I was being selfish. Driven by doubts and worry, I needed to be a bit more, a bit more... something... than I was, but I didn't know what.

Bob poured coffee from the cafetière. After so many years he knew how I liked it, unreasonably strong with hot milk, and more than enough so I could top up my mug. I tried to explain my conflicting thoughts and worries. 'How did you know E wouldn't hit you?'

The Governors' Conference, that annual beano of prison supremos, the event Bob was careering towards with a fanciful optimism, would never, could never, accept this as evidence of any change, could they? What were the officers thinking? Was E just a one off? How often would Bob see him? What did the psychologists think? I was riven with unanswerable anxiety after anxiety. I knew if we were to do this, I would need to live with the uncomfortably difficult possibility of never knowing with certainty what the outcome might be. Did I even know if I wanted to follow the journey that Bob had offered E? I was beginning to realise as well just how enormous was Bob's need for me to see, and talk through, the very guts of what he was attempting. *What was it he'd once said with a real yearning, a real meaning surrounding the impossible cliché? 'Follow me to the ends of the earth and back again.' Well maybe the dungeons of Parkhurst qualified! The dungeons of men's minds even! Even if I did, how could I do it?*

A trickle of excitement beset me. I didn't do boredom, and this wouldn't be boring. This was a surreal, and rare opportunity to witness a colossally important experiment. If it worked, maybe I could develop training programmes. *Would E face his fears?* I really didn't know. *And would Bob make it past the six months that the most optimistic of our gravely-worrying professional friends predicted?*

I felt fragmented. This glimpse into despair and hope was disturbing. It wasn't a particularly cold evening, but I remember feeling a chill and got up to poke the fire; a welcome bit of normality. We looked at each other. The relentless clarity of what I had seen couldn't be avoided with any amount of nice coffee or crackling logs. I heard the misery of the world clutching at me through the northern tones of E's voice. 'Well it was me mum, she used to batter me as a child.' There was hopeless, defeated grief in this big man's flat tones. As I had listened, I had seen a little boy, immersed in casual, meaningless brutality—no escape, no future, just an endless, fearful present. 'Come here I want to thrash you.'

Bob's gaze reflected not only E's pain, but that of his victims: there was not even a gossamer-thin membrane protecting Bob from the pain of all this understanding. Curiously, I was reminded of albinos who, devoid of protective skin colour, always knew the full force of the sun's light. 'Trust is a two-way thing', Bob was to tell me later, 'if I am asking E to face it, then I have to be able to.' His was an understanding only to be borne because he knew how to help to vanquish the terrors, but I didn't know! Nervily jittery, I didn't know what could possibly protect Bob. I didn't know how he could not feel scared, *and if he was scared, how could he provide E with the confidence to face the brutality and terrors of his past?*

Searching for relief, I started to interrogate Bob.

'I saw the connection. E was certainly listening, but I felt scared of him, and wondered what he might do, did you?... What was he like at the beginning? How has he changed? How can you hear all the horrors and not get too upset?' Anxieties burbled out of me. I didn't know what I wanted Bob to say, or what could reassure me. It all seemed impossible, a foolish ideological dream—conquering evil with kind words.

Bob tried to reassure me. Somehow, he didn't seem to need any. 'Violence is always a fear reaction, and my job is to find, and defuse the fear.' I did understand, but bomb disposal! *Well... what skill... what careful probing...* 'Oh Bob, how can you do it? You must be scared.'

'I was a bit... that first time with E when he waved his arms about, he's a big lad... but I can read violence now, see the little clues... test things a bit. Gently does it. E is beginning to see his fears, and when he has conquered them, his violence will evaporate.' It was an entrancing thought, and those earlier words of mine floated back. *If you are right, it will work here, and if it will work here it will work anywhere.* In truth I too wanted to find out, and was becoming hooked into the endeavour, into following and supporting these journeys. Resting back on Bob's certainty, I began to think that I could anticipate the obstacles lying ahead. I was gaining confidence in our strength, and as Bob talked I was beginning to think a positive story could emerge in time for the Governors' Conference. I felt eager to see the next powerful conversation.

The poignancy of this little scene after so many years still has power to sear. I can see the strength of our youth, pulsating with resilience and optimism; time stretching out eternally. Not yet fifty, my skin able to accept the smooth browning of summer sun, I was trim, my hair almost golden as I laid back on Bob's shoulder in our gentle living room. Our internal worlds of thoughts, ideas, questions and anxieties were colliding gently, and starting to merge. I didn't know, and could hardly have anticipated, the ugly collisions that lay ahead of us. For now, there was institutional endorsement, and all within were flexing their different muscles in unknown ways. These were the days before prison numbers doubled, before the idea that 'risk' could be managed out of existence, and rehabilitation became subservient to security. There was still a slight whiff of the traditional governor, doctor, priest triumvirate, attending to the needs of the State, the Body and the Soul. A kindly paternalism which offered redemption and salvation.

Pride

I had noticed Governor John's pride in his officers, their uniforms, their discipline, their solidarity, their loyalty and their stiff white shirts, but above all his pride in Parkhurst and its still-lingering traditions. The Number One Governor had automatic membership of the Royal Yacht Club, and a mooring on the Medina estuary. Officers joined in cricket matches encircled by the sea on the exposed Bramble sands during the summer low tide. This was a time when deputy governors could indulge in silly horseplay. Bob tells of an incident when a particular deputy solemnly supervised prisoners hoovering what grass there was with ancient vacuum cleaners. 'It's all right, he was reputed to have said, they're not plugged in.'

As well as being the all-powerful 'Mr Big' within the prison, John saw himself as a superior type of social worker and counsellor to the men, many of whom he had known over years as they served their long sentences. Politically, it was a time of conservative grandees with reforming consciences, and John spoke their language of reform and rehabilitation. I remember his wide and confident grin as he told me how great it was to bump into Bob around the prison. *Was Bob,* I thought, *part of his credentials as a rehabilitation supremo? The subject of boasting at meetings in London with his political masters.* In any event, this was a little opportunity, a little gap for a liberal experiment. Bob needed to push on, and I wanted to see whether other prisoners would accept his approach. Never could anyone possibly have realised that this was no liberal experiment. It was a radically clashing innovation. That would challenge all within the prison system.

Paradoxically it was the dispensing officer behind the Happy Hatch who seemed to cause Bob the most early grief. I thought of how I had felt when entering into a new work culture, and meeting colleagues for the first time. Everything new, a fog of uneasy expectations slowly clearing as working relationships developed, subterranean careerist manoeuvring still opaque within my civilised university establishment. So, what could Bob expect in such an elemental institution as a prison? Staff operated 24/7 on constant alert for assaults, suicides, escapes, drugs, bullying, personal sleights, career advancement, easy shift rotas. All defended by starched shirts and seemingly correct demeanours. The dispensing officer, flexing the muscles of his authority had given early vent to this and the lurking fears that were part and parcel of an impossible job. Bob was respectfully trying to develop some engagement with all that he was attempting. Sadly, I could see that he was stunned by encounters with covert mutterings, stares, and invisible obstructions. Indeed, there seemed to be little protective 'halo' effect for Bob from some quarters.

And anger ...

Seizing this emotional nettle as he clattered round the kitchen rinsing newly sprouting mung beans in a large glass jar, Bob told me 'There is a lot of anger at me.' His words carved into me like a knife. *Was this the start of an impossible battle? How could Bob possibly survive with angry colleagues?*

'It is both personal and not personal', I said to Bob, and trying to make it understandable, went on, 'the officers know their jobs, they've been trained for it, been doing it for years. I can even hear their voices. "We know what prisoners need better than fucking jumped up doctors, and their bits of paper. Dr Bob doesn't even know what these evil bastards are capable of. What we have to put up with day in day out. The only way to keep them sorted is the happy pills. He's acting like a lunatic and has to be stopped".'

And then I thought of Bob engaging with these dangerous men, seeing the drugs preventing their ability to change, to think, to transform. My head hurt trying to construct the big picture out of all this, a seemingly unbridgeable gulf of beliefs, training, ideas, skills, and actions. I had always relied on my brains, and took pride in my academic abilities: the linking together of disparate entities, innovative thinking and problem solving, but what could I say, let alone do, that would solve this? I rubbed my head, yearning for an easy way out. I couldn't find it.

Interrupting these painful thoughts, Bob was incisive. 'I have access to the men, that's the important thing, officers' approval will come when prisoners change, and everyone feels safer.' Putting down the pan of potatoes he'd just drained, he turned round and hugged me. 'Don't worry it's exciting.' *Exciting, exciting? Nerve-wracking, stupid, ludicrous, impossible, preposterous, outrageous maybe, but exciting!* I pulled away and looked at this tall figure, calmly going about the immediate business of putting a meal together, certain he could bypass obstacles and manage to succeed where the whole of the judicial system was failing. *Some day job this, persistent low-grade tripwires of grumbling hostility.*

Suddenly I broke into a wave of exhausted mirth: 'We can always do three things before breakfast, the impossible just takes a bit longer!' And so, we grinned ourselves into agreement, because it was, of course, this quality of obdurate certainty and courage that had so enticed me to Bob in the first place. My mind fled back twenty-six years. Bob was batting a tennis ball into the net. I enjoyed being a better player than him, and I'm still not sure what amused the onlookers more, my winning shots against this lanky, enthusiastic man, or the kisses over the net between points. In any event, at one of these intersections he'd said, 'Let's get married.' Unremarkable perhaps, except we had only met three weeks before, and Bob had meant exactly that — let's get married in two weeks, the soonest a special licence allowed. I had negotiated for three weeks, two weeks being unreasonable!

I remembered too how, out of the calm and quiet of a Quaker meeting, we had simply stood and married each other. *Friends, I take this my Friend to be my husband...* In the Quaker way there were no priests nor registrars to marry us, to officiate, to pronounce our union. Our jointly declared commitment, witnessed before our gathered friends and relatives, was everything.

I stuffed logs into our welcoming wood-burner as we settled down to a comforting evening together. *Calm after, or before the storm,* I wondered. We were in a many-headed race. *Could Bob change E in time for the Governors' Conference? Could he gain the trust of the prisoners soon enough to begin his work? Could he influence the officers before the anger spread, and became corrosive enough to really hurt him?* I imagined the multitude of little ways officers who controlled the hidden workings of the prison could make Bob's work unsafe. The Bronson incident had already unnerved me, but maybe all the routine nastiness, the rumbling uncomfortable discontent, was an even greater challenge than a murder threat. Brooding anger was surely only awaiting another, similar catalyst. For the moment Bob had his vision to pursue, and my work back in Manchester called, defying any immediate involvement on my part, but this attempt to rationalise my life, to manage the compartmentalisation, was to become acutely challenged every time I engaged with Bob, and the extreme nature of what he was attempting.

CHAPTER 6

The Man in the Blue Jumper

'I think I am getting somewhere, what do you think? He's probably the most influential prisoner on the wing... certainly feared... if I can crack him, the others will follow. Officers like to be on the right side of him. What's more he's agreed to be filmed.'

It seemed the morning meetings frequently revolved around a gossipy obsession with the man in the blue jumper. He was thought to be behind every little incident going—'Oh, that'll be him alright'—somehow attributing to him a fearful power. This was more than important for Bob. The man in the blue jumper was a threat to the officers: the calming of him was therefore crucial to their acceptance of Bob, as well as the calming of the wing.

Yet another telephone conversation was pulling me back to an immersion in an improbable, impossible world. This time too I couldn't avoid the challenge that awaited my return to Bob, and our house with its gentle gaze to the sea. Settling again in the scratchy sofa beside him, I adjusted some extra cushions and looked at the ill-lit video film. It was the man in the blue jumper. He hadn't seemed that fearsome when, fixing my eyes, he'd asked me if I'd let Bob come. Intrigued now, I bent forward, as if nearness would gain me extra knowledge.

This wasn't what I'd anticipated. His eyes held no appeal nor understanding, a veil of detached wariness obscured the gaze he directed just above Bob's head. He was lounging back, if it were possible to call it that, seated as he was in one of those ugly, uncomfortable prison chairs with his arms crossed and head tilted upwards. He wasn't a particularly tall man, nor large like E, but he had a controlled, wound-up, angry presence. As he moved to clasp his hands behind his head with a slight rocking motion, there was menace. I could see scars, ligature marks, yellow fingers and felt sudden fear. The threat seemed immediate, and I found myself pressing the pause button, relieved this was, after all, only a flickering on-screen presence in front of me. *Had I been fooled by* his earlier appeal, and bouncy demeanour? Whatever ghastly thing had I agreed to? This group of men had murdered outside, and a number had gone on to kill inside.

Darkness

Standing, I looked out into the dark garden. A flash illuminated the trees briefly. Outside now, I watched the rhythmic pulse of the nearby lighthouse as it flashed across the garden every ten seconds. *Curious that the light is there, flashing away all the time, but can only be seen at night. What surreal analogy is this,* I wondered, as my mind drew back to the image I was watching: *What possible light was there to be seen?* I saw only a man unbounded by compassion, an island remote and distant, surrounded by oh such heavy darkness. 'The impossible just takes a little longer', I muttered loudly. Caustic, and angry, I wasn't laughing this time. *Was this it then, our experiment ending before it had begun? Stupid risks. Stupid peril. Stupid work. Don't mess with me was the undoubted signal, but that was just what Bob was requesting of the man in the blue jumper—an invitation to mess with his head, his thoughts, his sense of self, his past, his traumas, his actions. The bargain was the goal of transformation, but did the man in the blue jumper want it, let alone think it in any way achievable? What was Bob seeing that I didn't?*

Banging the door shut, I entered our cozy room and stared at the still frozen figure on the screen. Bob was worried and upset, not about the man in the blue jumper, but about me, and it was true, I was hurting. 'It's not as bad as you are thinking, it's alright. Look, if it upsets you, don't watch it. I know what I am doing.' *But did he? This had never been done before. How can he be so certain?* I had doubts that hurt us both. Maybe I was being unreasonably fearful.

'Okay, okay, I will watch it, but you'll have to tell me what you were thinking.' I heard my loud, impatient voice and felt a twang of shame. Here was Bob, bravely tackling the most intractable of psychiatric problems in arguably the hardest, and least supportive of working environments, wanting my support and my encouragement, and all I could do was whinge about the risk. 'Sorry, I just need to know. Let's start again.'

Bob's voice begins, conversational and calmly inviting. 'I am looking for fear and anger from childhood, have you got any?' This time I tried to really see.

Suddenly the man in the blue jumper slumps into a softer shape, his head lowers, and he gazes sideways, as if searching a far horizon. Then, with quiet, measured deliberation he begins. His voice quiet, at odds with the evil he is describing, an endless film of gruesome horrors, playing on and on and on ... Bob listens, unflinching, bearing with him this unexamined knowledge as it staggers to a stop. 'It's not happening now, you are an adult.'

There is a long, too long silence. I want Bob to hug him and say, 'It's alright now', but instead he waits for the adult in front of him to emerge, to respond. Looking straight at Bob, the man in the blue jumper says, 'It's incredible to think, but it's like you said, I am a grown man, and still feel a frightened two-year-old. I am still scared to death of him. Scared it can all happen again, even though I can snap him in two with my bare hands.'

The anger welled out from a pit of deepest rage and fear. I didn't doubt his chilling capacity for harm. It was this that Bob was working hard to defuse, learning to construct the levers of trust.

'What did you see in him, how did you get him to trust you with his deepest fears?'

'I saw a struggling, shrunken young man in a lot of pain, who could have frightened me, but chose not to.'

'But the trust, what about that?'

'I told him the truth, what happens to your feelings when you're brutalised as a child. He thought I was a mind-reader at first.'

This video wasn't showing their first perilous encounter, when, against everything this man had ever experienced, Bob had succeeded in gaining a foothold of trust. I imagined what it must have felt like, the courage, the daring on both sides, like stepping over a cliff edge, trusting that it was soft sand, and no more than inches deep, rather than a precipitous fall to cruel rocks. What I was seeing was many sessions later. By trusting Bob to film this, the man in the blue jumper was granting the conversation an independent power and value, *but did he know this,* I wondered. *Could he, would he, ever transform sufficiently to talk about it, to add his informed voice in aid of Bob's endeavour?*

I came to think that for me this was the real start. The intensity of events was pulling me along. Any plans I had for gentle pauses and a quiet, careful regrouping were disappearing.

CHAPTER 7

A Hopeful Time

John's eagerness to showcase himself and Parkhurst at the upcoming Governors' Conference cast a mighty glow over Bob's activities. In these early days Bob never doubted he would be able to present a transformative account of how to work with violent disturbed prisoners, and John's need for this success story meant an aura of approval clung to Bob. That this was akin to a sprinkling of stardust in such an absurdly hierarchical institution Bob scarcely noticed, so focused was his intent, but John noticed, and was pained by Bob's lack of deference and acknowledgement of his status. This was something he couldn't insist on, for he traded on being benign and non-hierarchical, and Bob was even matching him in jokey good humour, for heaven's sake — this was his own, carefully honed, prison trademark persona.

When you are top of the tree any gesture of equality is illusory. Like the Queen saying, 'Call me Liz', it's not actually real; only a dismantling of the entire edifice can achieve that. And so, Bob cleaved his way through these currents, undercurrents and toxic eddies, choosing to not even see the encompassing tree, let alone its glowering extent, its branches, roots, and height stretching far beyond the Parkhurst prison estate. Later he was to say, 'I was far too busy... too much of a bother to notice.'

Maybe here lay the real seeds of the betrayals to come, but for the moment all was well, and I too so much wanted to dispel the lurking doubts, to stop my spiralling mesh of thought; too clever, too academic, too sharp, too anxious, my mind seemed incapable of stopping itself. It was left to a daft pigeon to provide me with my first reassuring sense that Bob was starting to control this new life. I watched as he carried some old, battered chicken wire up from the bottom of the garden. We had added it to our removal load in the fond belief that maybe we would keep chickens again, but by now it was a misshapen mass entwined with couch grass, and Bob was having difficulty keeping it from springing apart. It was an ugly bit of wire no doubt!

'What are you doing with that?'

'It's to keep the pigeon out.'

'What pigeon? What are you talking about?'

I learnt that a pigeon was in the habit of breaking into Bob's office cell. The heating was antiquated and inflexible, much like the prison itself. On all the time, the office was hot, stuffy and the opposite of fresh. Bob had to push his hand between the thick internal bars to open the window. Hence the daft pigeon's opportunity to poke his way in and flutter around dropping mess on table and chair, an intrusion as obvious as it was unwelcome. However, Bob could sort this one: the netting was waved through security by what I imagined were quietly amused officers and secured across the window. Henceforth the pigeon would mess elsewhere.

The Governors' Conference was now the immediate concern. By employing Bob, and by granting permission to film therapy with those deemed irredeemably bad, as well as mad, John had glued himself into a project he now had to show was a clever and successful managerial innovation. Stuck with goals perilously beyond any imaginings of headquarters' mandated targets, the stakes were absurdly high. It was an almost fanciful challenge. The conference was in October, two short months away, and only three months from the start of therapy with E. Bob had to show he could do it. Neither man, both being naïve and unreal in their own super-confident ways, could possibly forgo their challenges: Bob, to conquering the most difficult of all therapy, and John to be the youngest, most successful reforming prison governor ever.

The big man in small shorts had to change, had to respond, had to have courage. Not one person anywhere would have taken a bet on this; no officer, no counsellor, no prisoner, no psychologist, no teacher, no priest — certainly no psychiatrist. Antisocial personality disorders were considered untreatable: a 'disorder of personality' people were born with, an overweening medical take on the 'born evil' mantra. The best that could be hoped for was that in old age the condition would somehow 'burn out' as decrepitude overtook the individual.

Just a few years later, an even more hopeless diagnosis was to be born out of the entrails of an angry Home Office and Criminal Justice System. Reacting to the tragedy of the Michael Stone case of 1996 in which the authorities failed to act before he killed a mother, her young daughter and dog (injuring a second daughter), 'dangerous severe personality disorder' had to be spotted, and those given the label locked away pre-emptively if possible. Reflecting on all this now, it seems so bizarrely impossible that this moment of ours could ever have happened: a moment when these dangerously lost men were offered change, when the psychiatric system was confronted with a treatment, and the punitive nature of the justice system was challenged. The platform, the opportunity and the work lay ahead. I was infected by Bob's enthusiasm, the gripping nature of the need, and lulled by the seeming encouragement of the system.

The Big Man: my second encounter

And so it was that I came to look at the next video of E and tried not to feel fearful for this too-magnificently ambitious project. He was younger than I, but a mantle of lifelong despair sheathed his skin. There was a blank graininess, each pore, each cell of each pore seemed filled with a detached hopelessness. Instead of the joyful colliding of cells intent on growth, on life, these cells had given up. *No joy here, mate*, I imagined their helpless chat. I touched my own skin. It responded, yielded, still a bit pink from the spring sunshine.

'Well now E how've you been doing? What do you remember from last time?'

The normality of the cheerful enquiry sliced into the waiting air of this anything but normal space in the small cell. How could Bob ignore such brutal surroundings? From way back I recalled a textbook authoritatively mandating 'the core conditions for therapy' ... *gentle light, easy seating, fresh air, pleasant temperature, welcoming surroundings. Well, not textbook stuff then that I was watching, but maybe one still to be written...*

The large man stared and stared, shifting uneasily. Bob waited, his brown eyes anticipating and encouraging what he knew was so painful to even think. The silence lingered, more than was reasonable. Surely this was too hard—why didn't Bob say something? But then rubbing his eye with a finger, the response came: 'It's about me Mum, and how she used to batter me as a child.'

His words, flat and emotionless, struck the air like bullets. Who were they hurting? I saw the grossness of his fear as he glanced at Bob. His own words were terrifying him. His grubby, too-tight t-shirt moved slightly in a controlled gulp over his bulging frame. *What remorseless terrors were being inflicted on this small boy?* I felt a sudden shuddering of despair. *What comfort could Bob offer him, how could he make it better?*

He stared straight into my watching gaze. His eyes had disappeared into the darkness of his sleep-deprived flesh. I couldn't fathom them. Terror and trust were on a collision course. The words hovered between them. E scratched at some bristles by the side of his mouth. *What would come next, as they must surely dive into the chamber of horrors that was E's childhood? Would E, scared beyond endurance, crack with rage? How could they swim in the horror of it all, and somehow make it alright?* Careful warnings from seminars sprung into my mind ... *the dangers of re-traumatisation, too early disclosure, traumatic catharsis, acting-out, transference,* on-and-on they prattled through my too-receptive mind. There was no safety net for either of them in this comfortless environment.

Bob's challenge was calm, steady and totally unexpected: 'Yes but you are an adult, so why are you frightened? Why does it matter?'

Why does it matter, why does it matter? How could Bob be so stark, so blunt, so stupid? How could it not matter? He was leaping over the horror, ignoring the invitation to hear more. Was he really ignoring E, not listening to his pains and, sin of sins, was he not being empathic? Where was the comfort for E? My reaction was instant: thought and feeling merged in a mess of panic.

I saw the big man gaze at Bob. He didn't seem attacked, instead he was locked in thought, engaging in the challenge that Bob had put down. There was so much more to this than the words. *How had this bond been forged? How could E have begun to trust Bob with such certainty that he could begin to even think about his fear?*

I thought of when my own children were tiny, of their delicacy, their vulnerability and total helplessness; their trusting eyes, contentedly looking out with expectation of succour, of nourishment, of love. The big man never had this. His terrified baby brain had developed a miasma of terror toxically polluting each working thought. Bound in invisible chains of fear, he was paralysed. All free thought, choice, control, still unlearnt, he was on constant defensive high alert. A spring, only partially dampened by drugs, ready to explode with violence.

This all seemed an impossible task. My thoughts see-sawed. I saw the infant and felt anguish. I saw the man and felt fear. Maybe this really was too much. *How could such damage ever be repaired? Maybe we should retreat to safety. In any event, how could it be done in time for the conference? Even if these two brave* souls succeeded, how would sceptical, experience-battered Governors ever allow themselves to acknowledge such a fundamental challenge to their working practices, their assumptions?

Bob's words cut through my wandering feelings: 'Can you tell her you are an adult?'

'It would be nice to, wouldn't it...?' *Nice! Nice to be an adult, to claim the birthright of every baby as they grow into full adulthood.*

A piercing blue picture of tiny hyacinths in my garden, responding to a weedy rubble clearing, flashed through my mind. They were pushing themselves through to the spring sunshine, sometimes bending awkwardly in accommodation to a rough stone. *Was this what was going on? Bob providing the sun, and the big man glimpsing this, and tentatively starting on the journey through the rough ground to adulthood.* Bob was talking to the adult man, and it was the adult man responding—so Bob continued with his clearance mission:

'Would it? What advantage to you would it be, you telling her you are an adult?'

'Well, I could get on with my life couldn't I?'

'Could you? What would you say to her?'

'Well, I would say... "Mother, you can't hit me anymore, I am an adult."'

A flicker of fear crossed his face. He rubbed his nose. There was a cruel silence. *Surely Bob must reassure him now. 'No of course she can't, you are safe now'—surely that was needed?*

'And you believe that do you?' A stare, a silence, and then, amazingly, a breaking smile of knowing relief. The person facing him had earned his trust, because he not only knew the truth before even E did, but respected his otherwise humiliating, and secret feelings. Gathering his very self together, E took a huge breath and stated his emerging thoughts: 'Well, I partly do, and partly don't. I don't think I could say it to her though.'

A big pause as he drank in the import of the words... he couldn't tell his mother he was no longer a small child. With humiliating honesty, he was staring at Bob, grasping, almost gasping, for more relief. *What possible response could help? Maybe... 'Course you can, E, believe me it will be alright. Just try it. There's no need to be frightened, it's a false belief. You just need some practice. Give it a go.'*

But Bob, gloriously fearless, was still hunting down the engulfing fear:

'Why, what would happen to you if you told her you were an adult?'

'Well she might get up and clout me.'

E squirmed in the ugly plastic chair. I saw the white length of a scar on his large forehead as he bent his head downwards. The harsh painted brick wall glowered behind him. He was rocking ever so slightly from side-to-side, reaching for some long-gone elemental comfort. *Had Bob gone too far? Were these the signs of violence I'd been assured he was beginning to read?* A screaming *Stop!* pervaded my body, but then into the waiting moment came Bob's voice, confidently pulling the big man back into his adult self, into the reassurance of the present time. I heard the noise of my caged breath escaping as the interchange began, dissipating my tense alarm:

'Might she?'

'She might.'

'How old is she?'

'Eighty-five.'

'And she is going to do you an injury, is she?'

'Oh, she's still lively.'

'How big is she?'

'Five feet two inches.'

'And how big are you?'

'Six feet three and a half inches.'

Persistence

There had always been a penetrating persistence about Bob, I reflected. He was using it now, fearlessly inviting E to look at the truth, to say what he thought, however humiliatingly silly. And E, trusting, was following, responding, digging into his shuttered mind for the truth of his experience. Even now I find myself smiling. The conversation between these two powerful men was a careful fencing match. E parrying the truth. Bob landing oh-so-precisely gentle ripostes. Suddenly E leaned forward, pushing downward on the seat of his ugly chair. His face filled my watching gaze as he declared:

'Mother, you can't touch me, I am an adult. I would... I would say that.'

'And you believe that?'

'Partly.'

'You partly do, and partly don't?'

'Yes. I don't think I could say it to her. She thinks I am still in shorts.'

'Well, I believe you are an adult, and I believe she should be told.'

A grin crosses E's face, and Bob, laughing, says, 'Look her straight in the eye and say, "Look ma, I am an adult".'

E turns, stares to the side, grimly muddles the words, looks at Bob—a ghost of a grin flickers—then determinedly, he launches the words: 'Look ma, I am an adult. You can't touch me ever again, I've grown up, I haven't still got shorts on.'

I heard the strong confident tone of a man beginning to believe he could be in charge of himself. Then came a sudden, too-loud knock. Alert, E twisted in his chair, looking at the door. The careful moment was broken. There was of course a prison out there. Bob's words were reassuring: 'We'll conquer it. You're doing well. Thanks for coming along.' And so were E's: 'Of course…thanks.' His huge form filled the screen as he rose to shake Bob's hand, turned and left.

Too immersed in the intense, enclosed drama of the little screen, I didn't realise it was still only late-afternoon. The sun was promising a glorious sunset over the waiting sea. Bob too was waiting. He needed me to more than approve, to understand—to understand the cruel link between fear and violence. *Do I doubt it? Can I give Bob this reassurance? Is this really enough to explain—to convince hard, bruised Governors—that, at the heart of the fearsome violence they are charged with controlling and punishing, lies the trembling fear of tortured boys? And even more, that if this fear is dissolved, then violence evaporates?*

I gave Bob a hug. 'I am beginning to like E. He believes you.' I didn't know it then, but E was to be a template, the model against which I judged others' progress, and as I remember this I'm staring down at a page of neatly sprawling words on a sheet of lined foolscap, torn from a pad. It's a letter from E:

'I do know that you believe in me and I promised on the 11th Sept. 1991 I would never let you down. I haven't and I never shall.'

The deep, determined, underscoring of this letter shouted out at me. Trust remained, and was, a two-way thing on that September day, all those years ago.

CHAPTER 8

A Swimming Party

My sparky friend and John crashed into the kitchen shouting cheerily. Jolted out of my musings, I went to greet them. Faded towels were in a roll under their arms. 'How about a swim?' grinned an impish John, his hair bobbing and nodding as he strode through the kitchen and out into the garden. Bob and my friend followed, and I could hear their animated chatty laughter. Wanting, needing some time, I said 'You all go on ahead, I'll just shove some supper in the oven.' As their voices faded down the steep path to the sea I went outside. There was a lustrous stillness in the air. The sinking sun had tinged the sky with swirls of pink and grey. A little light, I knew, came into the prison cells, but not enough to prevent the harsh fluorescent tubes from being on all the time, Bob had told me, and of course, no moonlight could ever penetrate through the nighttime floodlights.

I shivered and turned to my culinary task, a chicken. *A bit more tasty because it's organic and was allowed to peck and eat and run about freely,* I hoped. Anyway, I stuffed it with three lemons sliced in half, and smeared it in honey. The honey made the skin a soft crunchy brown, and the lemons, well I love lemons, and always hoped for a lemony infused taste. We had kept chickens in our northern home. John and my sparky friend had been the recipients of the redundant hen house and galvanised hopper. I recalled, with not quite amusement, the time that John had discussed with Bob how to kill a chicken. It was I think a too-noisy cockerel. Bob had told him you hold it upside-down by its legs — mesmerised, it remains absolutely still — you then take its neck and twist it. The chicken dies instantly. As a child he'd often seen it done, it was quick and painless, he'd even done it himself.

We had all trooped out to the yard to watch. John, taking up the challenge with a confident bravado, seized the chicken and, the flapping stilled, tentatively yanked its neck. The chicken had squawked and flapped. Then a desperate John, tugging at the scrawny neck, managed to pull the head right off. It's true headless chickens can still run about. The residual nerves kept this one bloodily, nonsensically running. We had all responded with hysterical amusement, but I remember wondering uneasily why he hadn't just dropped the chicken, and why he preferred to pursue a bloody course with inadequate skills? He just couldn't put it down and let it run away, there was never going to be an easy way out for the chicken or John. Recalling it now, I can see how shocked we all were, and I can see too how our affection for John prevented us acknowledging that it really was bizarre macho posturing.

No wonder I had felt uneasy. After shoving the meal into the oven, I felt cross, beleaguered and scratchily irritated as I set off down the path to join our jolly friends. Nearing the sea whoops of splashing joy floated towards me on the evening air. *Oh, this is lovely... whatever the wider looming questions.* It *was* lovely, my doubting head calmed as I met the rhythmic waves.

The Governors' Conference

Walking back up the hill, the men were elated. Full of the power of their work, they were confident and animated. The Governor pleased with his capture of a tame psychiatrist, was eager to display the results, and the Psychiatrist, basking in unusual encouragement, was eager to demonstrate his breakthrough. I hoped this jollity, this friendship would survive the conference.

This was to be at a hotel in a sometime-genteel watering hole on the South coast of England. Out of season, it would still be warm, unlike the chill and damp of the North. I had seen pictures of iconic palm trees in blue-skied brochures. 'What are you going to wear?' was my parting comment as I once more started my journey back to Manchester, and work. I really didn't know the dress code for this most status conscious gathering, but I did know that Bob's idea of smart casual, an eclectic mix of clothes favouring bright colours, and padded warmth, was undoubtedly tricky. 'Just wear your prison suit with a white shirt', I advised, 'you can use the new ones we've just bought.' Bob, gloriously indifferent to matters sartorial, acquiesced. I found myself thinking, *The more radical the message, the more sober the suit: an agreed uniform of power only available to men.*

I thought of my own difficulties in addressing conferences. Apart from the content, always a problematic negotiation. There were the endless personal presentation questions: *Trousers? Skirt? Heels? Colours? Fashionable? Dowdy? Expensive? Modest? Hairstyle? Hair colour?* But for men, merely tie or not? I realise I still don't know these sartorial messages, and actually love Bob's supreme indifference to these small but irritating matters. Whatever, I would have to sort his shirt-maintenance issues at some point, but for now this would suffice, and I went back to Manchester confident he would look every inch a consultant psychiatrist. He had the height for a suit, and an engaging, well-defined face. I hoped he would trim his beard before he left.

Having driven from the island in John's battered old estate, they arrived at the venue. Neither man was ever short of words to describe the importance of his work, and it must have been one of the most surreal conversations ever that they hurled at each other as they travelled along the South coast's ever-clogged roads; a sparring froth of escapes, murders, kidnaps, violence, trauma, reform, rehabilitation, transformation, causation, change, evil. I'd seen how supercharged they could be and were. On a feeding frenzy of ideas, hopes, and ambitions, as John's latent idealism was fed by Bob's clarity and integrity of purpose, and Bob's intellectual ambition was fed in turn by John's apparent agreement.

As John eagerly glad-handed his way around the hall full of his peers, and crucially, a dose of superiors, a message came over the waiting loudspeakers. 'The police would like to see the owner of vehicle number such-and-such…' Governor John had not only parked in the wrong place, but the tyre treads were illegal. Faced with his status, and the importance of the conference delegates, the police merely reminded him to 'Move the car and get it fixed, Sir', a carefully laughing John had told Bob and those all around. However, as the time for their address to Conference arrived, John simply disappeared. Billed as a joint effort, Bob's success would be John's glory, but John, realising at last the radical challenge Bob was about to unveil, absented himself. Bob was on his own as he stood to face the sea of sceptics, kindly ready to give him an amused hearing. They knew John as a bit of a joker, and must have been anticipating some relief from the overload of the weighty programme.

Bob starts: 'Violence is the long-term effect of trauma in childhood. Trauma results in frozen terror. Dissolve the terror, and the violence evaporates. He turns to the video camera. 'E has agreed to let me show you how he is managing to overcome his terror and the effect it has on him.'

And then the button pressed, E crashes into the comfortable imaginings of that comfortable audience in that oh-so comfortable seaside resort. His big frame stares out. 'It's about me mum and how she used to batter me as a child.' It's authentic, visceral, true. The audience, of course, isn't: there are careers, positions, protocols, politics, and the public to attend to. Alarmingly honest, the presentation is greeted with total silence, tinged with covert respect.

Back home, Bob couldn't recall a single question being asked, but circulating in the bar afterwards he'd caught snatches of uneasy banter. 'I'd better watch what I do to my kids then.' The private emotional space, a space we all inhabit, had collided with the public space of ordered, regulated, mandated action. It had been the opposite of comfortable for this audience of supreme regulators.

Nevertheless, I did know it had been a presentation which couldn't be forgotten, either by me or any of that tightly corralled audience. When next I returned to our island home I hugged Bob tightly, and so hoped the seeds of an alternative, sown there in that South coast conference room, would begin to blossom. Bob remained, as it seemed to me, bizarrely exultant. His passionate endeavour to discover what lies behind violence was succeeding. He had found the truth of it, and he had shown it. That was what truly excited and supported him. Plaudits, acclamation, recognition, career, money, were never his concern. Indeed, I reflected. *If they were, these toxic motivators would have strangled both his focus and ambition.*

I managed to remain comfortably unaware of just where such a noble passion for showing the truth could lead, and Bob, indifferent to the lack of acclamation, was charging on to the next challenge: 'Must get to see X.' X was the shadowy, scrawny, unkempt figure confined in a caged cell in the optimistically named Hospital Wing.

I couldn't let my worry go, as an unbearable image beset me, of Bob standing in that seaside hotel, tall, clear, sure, and coherent. Not only was he giving an explanation for murderous rage, but incredibly the path for undoing it. *And for this to be ignored— How could he possibly stand it? Why didn't they realise, see what they had got in front of them? Prisons are stuffed with dysfunctional misery, didn't they ever ask why?!* I was angry and bothered. Too upset to be aware of my fear, I was holding out for the balm of acclamation, of praise.

I still hadn't decided to leave my job. I was getting acclamation of sorts in Manchester. *What would I do? How much did I need it? I can't justify myself through Bob's work, or can I?* That was never the plan, but Bob couldn't do it without me. *So what's my role? And the money...* My job was secure, Bob's wasn't, indeed he hadn't even got a contract. I couldn't then have possibly known just how crucially helpful this chaotic omission by the Prison Service was to be. I was caught in a mesh of clashing desires: an old life of familiar friends, wrought out of politics, social action and family, a life of self-confidence, wrought out of academic study and work. In a sudden moment of joy, striding through the campus into work, I touched the bark of carefully-planted saplings. A light breeze echoed through their leaves.

When I returned to the island for my next weekend visit these unresolved thoughts were still flying through my head. Bob, well Bob was still musing about X. 'X. Now that's really a challenge.'

Unaware of my turmoil, he wasn't even slightly bothered by any lack of acclamation from conventional authority, whether it be his profession, the Prison Service or Whitehall mandarins. He was troubled only about his own competence, whether his skill was adequate, his knowledge sufficient. Feedback from the men, that was all that mattered to him as he progressed his explorations into the truth of the matter. Painful strategic and political considerations he had neither the time nor inclination to pursue. My stomach clenched in a twisting and sudden revolt. 'Why aren't you bothered?' 'I'm absolutely bothered!' 'X is a challenge, but what about me? I'm a challenge, my bloody job's a challenge!' This blast of confused rage hurled towards a startled Bob, was shocking to us both. We paused for a long, long moment.

'Give me a hug', I said shakily.

'You know I love you beyond measure', said Bob.

As his arms strong and long folded tightly around me, I considered my angry worries. In the kitchen of this island home of ours I had recently hung a circular mirror which reflected a view of the sea and waving trees. It had hung in the small hall of my childhood home, a mirror from the 1940s, its roundness moderated by angled cuts along its rim. I liked it. Now it was reflecting me as I gazed over Bob's shoulder. *What was I seeing? I couldn't tell. Was I stuck in the foothills of a mountainous journey, never to reach the uplands? Bob was climbing his crags with relish.*

Remembering this struggle now, I realise that, difficult as it was, I was always going to engage in the battle. I could never have walked away. Bob's vision, courage, clarity, E's bravery in facing the truth and the silent contract I had made with the man in the blue jumper when I entered C-Wing that very first time were dragging me on. I know too that it was more than this. The competing primacy of thoughts and emotions, rationality versus passion, had always engaged my intellectual life. My university studies had left me growling at mandated philosophical texts, which determinedly placed these living issues in separate, sealed silos; dry logic excluding any attempt at merger.

And this battlefield was here, in all its raw immediacy: precise rational logic was justifying, cloaking, restraining, hiding, a brute emotionality, an emotionality that produced carefully organized protocols of punishment, revenge, hatred, deterrence, disgust, fear and despair. I thought with a tiny pang of the carefully purchased dark blue chairs patiently waiting in my office up North. They were relaxingly low and padded, grouped around an encouraging coffee table. And then the challenge of those oh-so-starkly uncomfortable prison chairs, waiting motionless in that despairing harsh prison light. Thus engaged the battle of the chairs. The newly expectant dark blue was never going to win. They still had their position, their importance, their future. The ill-matched, ugly, un-self-regarding prison chairs had none.

Early retirement

So, I returned to a disbelieving university and enquired about early retirement. It wouldn't be a great deal as I had child-rearing gaps, but yes, it was available once I reached fifty if the institution agreed, which they did in a surprisingly nonchalant manner. Hurt and distressed at this apparent lack of regard for me and the work I loved, into which I had poured so much thought and energy, I was later to learn through the tears of a stunned boss that no-one had believed me. They had thought I was bluffing, manoeuvring, looking for advancement, and that I couldn't, or wouldn't possibly leave. And it was true. I obviously enjoyed my work. It was nationally regarded. I was still planning projects, and new funding, and how were they to know I always meant what I said? *How indeed?*

Holding the small bottle of scent I had been given during that last tearful encounter, I get a whiff of emotive fragrance and reflect on the idiotic lack of trust that helped me to leave, and an institution to fund the loss of a valued employee. *They actually paid me to go away when they wanted to keep me. If I had been trusted, ways would have been found to try and keep me, making my struggle exquisitely harder.* I remember my dismay, my disbelief, almost rage at knowing I hadn't been believed, of knowing my words, my very self had been discounted. And I hear the echo of those words of E's: *I have told you the truth, haven't I? You do believe me, don't you?*

Parkhurst was to offer a brutally live case study, a piercing challenge to understanding the consequences of trust and mistrust...

CHAPTER 9

A Barbecue

And now it was springtime up North. The catkins were beginning to shake in every gentle breeze, and masses of yellow, gold and papery white daffodils filled our daughter's flat as we prepared to celebrate her wedding. John and my sparky friend came too, John flamboyant in the striped blazer he had worn at his own wedding only a few months before. I was fifty. It was time to move on. Driving South to join Bob after the close of the summer term, I felt some glorious liberating hope, and found myself singing *I am going where the sun shines brightly, I am going where the sky is blue…*

There was to be a barbecue on C-Wing, and I was invited, Bob announced. The men were looking forward to seeing me again. A barbecue! Images of gardens awash with summer colour, hot sun, and smells of burning charcoal. *Is my hotdog ready yet?* Sizzling sausages, hamburgers, lamb chops and eager children flooded my mind. *A summer evening progresses.* Easy confidences and anecdotes are exchanged, along with the offerings of beer and cold white wine. *But what could I expect of a C-Wing barbecue?!* I felt an unease, almost a foreboding, as I pictured the paradox.

Spreading humanity

John was trying to spread a leavening of humanity, a nod to a normal happy life of fellowship into these lives, whose own futures, as well as those of their victims, had been obliterated. John was easy to caricature with his huge grin, glasses and mass of hair. He was becoming the butt of many a cartoon, and some found their way onto the walls of his downstairs loo. The *Daily Mail* reserved an especial animosity for his particular brand of liberal gestures. They were easy targets. *A barbecue? What kind of cushy holiday camp was this? A murderer's reward while decent folk slaved.*

I had bought this summer dress in Manchester. It was a type of loose seersucker cotton, plain and with long with sleeves, a dropped waist and belt I never used. I still have it, and like its faded yellow. Today, I suppose it might be called urban shabby chic, with a touch of retro. The cotton is thinning and it needs some stitches to keep it going, but back then it was just a comfortable cotton summer dress with buttons; gentle enough for an outing to a maximum-security prison and the delights of a barbecue.

This time an officer met us at the gate and guided us courteously through the mess of wire enclosures and locked gates. In the distance I saw the still carefully trimmed hedge, its little pink flowers blooming even more strongly in the summer sun, and then, unlocking the final gate we were ushered politely into the C-Wing compound. A few of those ugly prison chairs were dotted around on cracked concrete, struggling to maintain a proper balance as the whole area was on a slope. The surrounding wire fences were tall, very tall, over twenty feet I judged, and strung up on high, crisscrossing the open view to the sky, were steel cables. 'To stop helicopter escapes', I was told.

It was open, open to the air, open to the sky. We were outdoors, but the space was so tightly shackled, so bound that all of that meaning had fled. It was an ugly grey and colourless sight I gazed at, except for tiny scraps of green where the odd brave weed had pushed its way through the concrete cracks. Officers in short-sleeved white shirts were purposefully standing with their backs to the fence at what I assumed were strategic locations. A couple of them were tending the barbecue, embarrassedly poking sizzling sausages on an industrial-size grill. *Made out of half an old steel oil drum,* I thought.

And then there were the men. I had supposed that outdoors it would all feel more normal, less trapped, less frightening, but no. They were, and I was, inside a huge wire mesh cage. All of us watched by flat-faced keepers, concealing boredom, anger, pity, I couldn't tell. To my immediate gaze the men seemed shrunken, I supposed in comparison to the unnaturally tall fencing, even thin Little K, the man who'd busily offered me those sadly sparkle less buns at the tea party, seemed particularly withered, weak orange squash in plastic cups no substitute for his ever-present pint mug of six-bag tea. Remembering this scene now, knowing what I do, I can scarcely bear to look. Back then my gaze was suffused with hope, that soothing, confident anticipation of work to be done;

otherwise the screaming reality of it must surely have kicked me flat. Older now, I look back in some awe at the resilience of hope.

As we entered, a barely visible faint alertness enveloped this carefully delineated collection of men. The officers stiffening whilst the meandering prisoners gave glancing looks. The men were idling, moving around with no seeming purpose, each in his own space. This party was being used as an opportunity, afforded by a large compound, *not* to get together. The careful accommodation between watched and watching was in danger of dissolving as Bob smiled, wanting to introduce me to officer and prisoner alike. E, spotting us, strode up, defying the lurking conventions of this most curious of parties. 'How are you doing, Sue?' he said, proffering a limp flabby white roll enfolding a thick, charred sausage. From somewhere I recalled that prison dogs had a larger feeding allowance than the men, statistics I had hoped weren't true but now, as I accepted E's offering, I could well believe it.

As E and Bob joked together, I noticed to my right, nearer to the barbecue and within range of the officers, a small group of men clustered around a chair. On the chair was a tiny round elderly woman. I learnt later she was a prison visitor, a volunteer who for many years had been visiting prisoners who were totally cut off from family and friends. I was surprised to see that the man in the blue jumper was seemingly in charge of the jostling group, invisibly reserving access to a precious resource. *Peter Pans, still in Gruesome Land responding to the mothering they never had.*

I couldn't see the thin man who'd told me about the gallows. Apparently, he'd refused to leave his cell. Remembering the painful, careful mispronunciation of words he'd never heard spoken, I sadly understood the beckoning safety of a cell. Then John clashed through the metal gate in a flurry of important grins, jokes and smiles. Leaving his accompanying officer to secure the gate, he bounced his way towards us, nonchalantly picking up a sausage on the way. He was carefully not put out to see me, I noticed, but it was clear he hadn't expected to see me *there*. *There are permissions, then, that don't go through the Number One Governor,* I thought, glancing over to the correct but kindly-looking officer who had met us at the gate.

'Enjoying yourself?' John grinned meaningfully, and then, talking about my sparky friend, said, 'She would have come if she'd known you were going to be here.' So that was it. An opportunity to display their girls to the men, to compete in liberal sociability. Bob missing all this, smiled and said, 'Good thing to do this, John.' But it wasn't liberal sociability I was engaged in. It was more intense than that. There seemed to be an invisible, taut connection between Bob and the circling men. I was part of that connection. I was Bob's hinterland. If it was sound, then maybe Bob was. So it was that I found myself in the strangest of interview situations.

The man in the blue jumper scurried up, clearly well-used to talking with John. Keen to help Bob, he proudly informed John of the good work Bob was doing. The men were benefiting, the unit had had no alarm bells rung. John stiffened and laughed uneasily. 'He's not a one man show you know' and moved away to talk to the old lady. Bob continued to chat to the man in the blue jumper, who was so pleased with his gift to Bob: praise from arguably the most powerful and dangerous man on C-Wing to the most important man in his bounded universe.

The sun still shone, the barbecue still sizzled, the officers still watched. There was nothing to indicate that this was the watershed moment it proved to be. True, I felt a tingle of unease at John's abrupt departure, but this soon dissipated as a young prisoner breaking away from his thoughts came hesitantly towards us.

'Hello S, this is my wife, Sue.' As I shook his hand his brown eyes flickered over me. He was curly-haired and so young, with the look of an unformed teenager, life still to present itself. *What hideous path had led him here?* My heart wrenched at the solidity he found in Bob, a still moment in all his horrors, he seemed to steady in his presence. *Like quietening a colt,* I almost thought. Many years later I was to meet him again in another strange and unforeseen encounter, but as of now he was the baby of the wing.

Another man now presented himself. I had noticed his snake-like progression around the perimeter of the compound. He was lanky, with long hair waving around his shoulders. This time any connection was oblique, obscured by what fears I couldn't tell. Something drew him towards us, then he skittered off, muttering something to an officer who nodded, unlocked the gate, and escorted him back to the wing. He finally contrived to be removed from the wing entirely, after angrily denying there was anything wrong with his childhood. I later found out, from his sad little letter of confession to Bob, that he'd been too terrified of the awful truth to confront it.

A Barbecue

So, there I was, the prison psychiatrist's wife. Had I passed the interviews? I felt wrung-out, exhausted, tired of being so watched by both prisoners and officers alike in this so-carefully-non-watching way. I craved the normal air, I craved anonymity. *Was that the cruellest part of incarceration?* Squeezing Bob's hand I asked him, 'Have we done enough, can we go?'

'I want to introduce you to the officers first. It's nearly over. We'll need someone to take us to the gate.' Bob too needed to show me off, to gather additional approval from the officers if he could. I did my best, and indeed it was a task that had echoes of familiarity. I recalled trying to win over plumbing, welding, and engineering lecturers to the idea of staff training and development, and the scepticism with which my 'non job' was received, but this, this wasn't a game of muttering irrelevance. Security and safety were the looming levers behind every rule, every action. Even John's show of benign humanity was carefully corralled within the rules. This was a frightening place, in which dogmatic, mandated training gave a measure of reassurance to even the most inexperienced officer. *Was Bob making it harder or easier for them?* This was a conflicting question in this non-questioning environment. I sensed liking, suspicion, hostility, confusion and almost jealousy as I politely smiled and said 'Hello.'

Suddenly, pushing knowingly rudely into these polite introductions, came a short, fat man. Standing far too close he neither looked nor smelt clean. I shook his hand as he leered with a touch of menace-filled bravado. 'So you're the wife?' Bob quickly intervened. 'Yes, P this is Sue... Enjoying the barbecue?' This really was too up-close and personal. It scared me, challenged my liberal imaginings. I was glad the officers were around, but Bob was undisturbed. I realised he had a certainty of understanding, of purpose, that eluded me, but supported him.

'I'm glad I was there. E was pleased to see me, he has changed, hasn't he? John was a bit funny don't you think? Where was the CMO? I'd have thought some of the psychologists would've been there. I suppose I should have talked to my sparky friend about it, but she wouldn't've come anyway, not really her scene...' John could of course only order his officers to attend. Musing a bit I thought, *The professional ranks don't socialise with prisoners, it's something about keeping a proper distance, remaining objective, resisting ever-lurking dangers of manipulation...*

We chattered on in some relief. As we drove through the winding summer lanes the world seemed newly fresh, large and open. Looking back at that sunny barbecue afternoon, I realise now it foreshadowed and showcased all of what were to be the conflicting hallmarks of our years at Parkhurst: defeat and acceptance, rejection and support, acclamation and denigration, kindness and anger. We never knew what each day might bring. Nevertheless, that steady connection, the work with the prisoners, the only thing that counted for Bob, remained a constant.

'P scared me... how violent is he?'

'Don't worry about him, he makes a point of being offensive. His belly's huge. He once wedged a ruler under it and strutted round on display. Might be the drugs he's on doesn't help. He's still walking round me. Won't talk yet, but we'll get there. Talks about himself as "rubbish".'

'I'm not surprised, he was a walking dustbin, complete with smell!' Bob laughed, 'Yes I'll crack it though.' He was so clear, so confident. I saw the lifeline he was offering another lost boy, and felt like weeping. Instead, I squeezed his knee and said, 'Well done.'

Normality

And so we returned home to what I came to think of as our 'island fastness' and a bit of normality. Bob cooked the fish he delighted in obtaining fresh from the local fisherman, whose yellow boat dodged the waves in front of our watching windows. I wondered where this fish had been swimming that morning and with what anticipation of the day ahead. That second summer was a still novel time for me, of sunny warmth and murmuring sea. The sound of our clanging garden gate began to be more reassuring, but I still awaited the latest revelations with a touch of foreboding I hoped would somehow, sometime, just vanish. A glimpse of slugs disappearing, collapsing into the ground on contact with salt, flashed into my memory. *But where was the magic salt that could collapse all my lurking anxieties, and their grumbling companion irritation, that useless irritation I keep trying to dissipate?*

CHAPTER 10

The Hospital Wing

There was news from the Hospital Wing. Bob had connected with X, that shadowy, bearded figure in the improvised cage. A spot of socialisation was being tried by the CMO. So the heavy metal door to X's cell had been locked back, leaving only the barred gate. It reminded Bob of the bars in Marshalsea Debtors' Prison, a one-time home for Charles Dickens' father. We had seen them, displayed in the Dickens Museum. The ones Bob was to stare so intently through didn't have that bleak blackness, they were painted in cream gloss and a bit chipped. I suppose it helped, and somewhat idly wondered if they were of the same vintage, they were built to last, after all. I wondered too about the decorator, brush in hand, who must surely have missed out on the normal acclamation for his work: *What a difference, that's so much better!*

However, welded onto this particular gate was a dense, tight, grey wire mesh, I supposed to prevent any thrusting through of hands. *No need then for any Zoo-like notices, 'Danger, don't feed the animals.'* Particularly as there was a large slot with a metal flap at the bottom of the door through which a tray of food could be pushed. These domestic details escaped Bob, and it was only when I read some technical specifications I realised the extent of this confinement, and the amount of detailed thought, work, and expense it all required.

The CMO, responding to Bob's careful request, and nonchalantly impressed by what he'd heard, had told X that Bob would be visiting the Hospital Wing. This was his chance, the longed-for opportunity to explore, to understand, to liberate. It was a beyond-reason challenge, to help this gruesome figure resolve the demons that had produced so much terror, a terror proportionate to the extreme incarceration he was experiencing: the prison too was frightened. It wasn't only the bars Bob had to see beyond. *How could he ignore this man's brutal capacity?* For me it was a chilling foreground, but I came to understand that for Bob it was this never-forgotten background, the compulsive driver of his work at Parkhurst. X was a vital benchmark, the most extreme of targets, against which his radical ideas about the cause, and cure for violence, could be refined, developed and proven. More than rare, it was indeed a unique laboratory for my dearest daffy one.

Now, so many years later, I wonder at how this came to be normal for us, merely after-work conversations, debriefings on the doings of the day. I had been pleased for Bob. Pleased! That my husband was standing in front of a serial killer, trying to start a therapeutic conversation through bars and mesh. Naïvely at first, I had supposed that both of them would be sitting down for this first encounter. But, no, Bob explained he wasn't allowed entry into X's cell and anyway, any chair in the cell was immovable, because of course, it was bolted down. 'Hi X, how are you doing?' was Bob's opening attempt at coaxing the hesitant, waiting figure to come forward, and stand before that solidly locked gate of bars and wire mesh. Bob is inches away from X; looking, connecting, and somehow managing to ignore the tight, grey wire barrier. He explained how he could just about maintain eye contact, but if either man moved, even slightly, then the bars got in the way. I imagined this surreal sight; a frozen tableau of necessity: static and still.

Childhood influences

Reporting the conversation to me, Bob had said to X, 'I am interested in looking at violence and childhood influences.' X merely said 'Oh' and a long pause followed then a strange elliptical conversation began. X said '... I have a friend who might be interested in what you do. How do you go about it? I could tell him.' Then Bob gently explained 'Well it's about fear and anger from childhood and how it affects what happens in adult life. It's about getting *your friend* to trust me to allow me to help him dissolve his fears.'

That evening as I listened, I was anxious. 'So how long did it go on? How did you leave it? Will you see him again? Were the officers watching?' Questions tumbled out of me, and then a visceral fear gripped as an unseen vision of X hit me, his hot breath besmirching that treasured face. 'What did he look like? Was he clean? Did his breath smell?' Bob laughed. He was delighted with his progress. 'You silly old thing...' he smiled. 'He's fine. Long hair. Long beard. Long face. Otherwise perfectly presentable. Just utter misery. I made a connection though, he talked indirectly. I need to see him in his cell. We'll steady away…'

'Oh Bob, what an ambition, to sit in a serial killer's cell!' I felt a sudden twinge of sympathy for that officer who had angrily declared, 'These animals are getting Harley Street treatment. My wife can't get it', and of course I could've been a Harley Street consultant's wife. *Bob has the charisma, the qualifications and a saleable authoritative charm.* It was a thought that thankfully never truly lodged. It was too far away from this pressing quest.

'But who was noticing, what did they think?' Bob laughed again, unconcerned. 'Don't think there was anyone around.'

X's particular cell, I learnt, was in a back corner of the first floor of the Hospital Wing. It was deliberately isolated. There were empty cells on either side. Most of the hospital prisoners were in cells on the ground floor where their medical state could be more easily checked, so this charged, this so-uniquely rare conversation had passed without notice. That Bob was being ignored was too strong a statement. He was an irrelevance. So little-noticed that it wasn't worth the trouble of dignifying him with a lack of recognition. That was to come later, though I clung to a suspicion that somehow the CMO knew, and was invisibly cheering Bob on. I wondered too if Bob's excluded pigeon ever visited. I was sure he'd get a welcome. *But maybe the privilege of fresh air was Bob's alone: the windows are a good foot behind the bars, and high up and small.*

It hurt to look at Bob. I knew he would be visiting X, even if the pigeon couldn't. Crying now, I couldn't tell either of us why. Maybe I was weeping for the seeming impossibility of it all. Multitudinous ideas, thoughts and visions kept prowling around. Sense battled with nonsense, whilst Bob, the opposite of distracted, was driven, strong and deliberate. He was forging a very new path.

'Cheer up, it's not as bad as all that!'

'Well it might be. I know you. You're going to go into that cell. How do you know he won't kill you too?'

'I know what I'm doing. I'll get his trust first. It's possible, really it is, but I can't do it without you. I need you to understand.'

'Understand! Understand! Of course I do, I understand too much! It's humanity and inhumanity, it's transformation or retribution, trust or suspicion… it's you against the prison, the officers, the psychologists, the psychiatrists, the prison system—the Home Office. No-one agrees with you.'

'That's a bit extreme. They will when I show them it's already a safer place.' I was instantly sorry. That was of course the vision, the ideal, I too shared. 'Even if it doesn't work it's right to try', I found myself saying.

We had ended up in the garden. It was starting to get dark. I shivered as a looming sense of doom enveloped me, along with the oncoming chill. Bob hugged me, and I found myself immersed in a memory: *9.25 in the morning in our sunlit garden, the recent eclipse of the sun just beginning, and we are waiting, watching, as the sun is slowly, remorselessly rendered black and lifeless by the moon; a chill accompanies the eerie darkness, and the birds fall silent, until the slow return of light and warmth as the blockading moon moves on its way. What dread events still eclipse X's light? How could Bob possibly reverse it?*

Putting the videotapes on record

'I hope he agrees to be taped', Bob said, 'it's such important stuff.' Ah... the tapes! The tapes that were to play such a dramatic part in our story. Ever since the Governors' Conference, Bob had been asking prisoners for their permission, obtaining written consents, and filming all the interactions he could. Cheaper by the dozens, he had kept himself more than supplied with pristine blank tapes. Stacked in his study they were patiently awaiting their time of importance. As they filled, they were given codes, dates and their own locked space. All those ephemeral words, glances, twitches, were accumulating, being captured before they drifted off into pale memories.

With a sudden practical foresight Bob had consulted an intellectual property lawyer as to the correct wording for the men's consent, and with an astonishing prescience also wrote a letter to John informing him he was now filming his work, and that he envisaged a time when it would be in the public interest for it to be televised. There was no response. In the blizzard of memos and directives that daily passed across John's desk, this one could surely be ignored as an overweening impossibility, but Bob persisted with a second memo requesting that it be sent further up the line to Prison Service headquarters. There in John's in tray it remained 'just a memo', forever unanswered, until its magnificent High Court appearance (of which more later). That all lay ahead of us, but now I was anxiously still entangled in understanding, still seeking the reassurance that Bob's work was considered important.

CHAPTER 11

The Guardian

Our first media exposure was accidental, through a casual conversation Bob happened to have. This was to be a constant backdrop to our years at Parkhurst, as the very name was a trigger, a name stuffed with meaning, an archetype of dread incarceration. Add in serial killers, psychiatry, therapy, transformation, and the mix became not only fascinating but compulsively magnetic for any journalist. The assumed public appetite for 'gore', as Bob termed it, was to clash fearfully with his determined efforts to inform, and to speak the truth. Despite all my big picture imaginings, I never got remotely close to anticipating its threatening end.

Melanie

Back then Melanie Phillips was a journalist on the *Guardian*, a newspaper I read most days, particularly enjoying its social and political comment. So, when Bob told me she wanted to come and talk about his work, I was familiar with her clever, well-argued and incisive opinion columns. 'She's a grown-up thinker, I'm sure she will understand your ideas. It'll be good to have them reported.'

'Yes, she wants a good chat. Should I invite her to lunch? She wants to see the men. I'll ask John to okay it. He'll be fine, he likes publicity.'

The following week Melanie came to lunch. She must have set off early from her London home. Bob met her at the ferry while I made a bean stew. I liked her. I liked the strong, serious conversation we all had. I liked her capacity to listen. I liked her directness.

'Does the stew have shellfish in it?'

'No…'

'Good.'

She will be able to position Bob's work accurately, I reflected. Ironically, she was the first, and only one, to see quite how much Bob's theories 'challenge opinion on both left and right.' Used to enjoying academic discourse, I was enthusiastic, chatty, totally unaware of how rare her journalistic honesty was, not to say her attitude to me. Unlike so many of the opportunistic commentators who were to follow, she listened deeply to me, despite a tinge of bafflement at my participation, and my presence, but of course, in all honesty, it must have been confusing. *Who was I? What was I? The prison psychiatrist's wife, code for 'invisible servant', or what?!* I too struggled with a label that denoted such unnoticed unimportance. Saying goodbye at the gate as they drove off to see John and the prisoners, a sudden lurch of unbidden frustration came powering in. Moodily I loaded the dishwasher. I'd have kicked the proverbial cat if we'd had one.

The visit had gone well, Bob informed me later that evening. John had shown her round and given the men permission to talk with her. E, and the man in the blue jumper were particularly keen. They had signed consents for what they said to be reported.

'That's good, they must have trusted her. What about their names?'

'No, they wanted their names to be left out, but they confirmed all we talked about.'

'What did you think of her?'

'I think it was worth talking to her. I think she gets it. Let's hope they print it.'

'Was John okay?'

'Yes, he likes being a progressive governor.'

Publication

The following Friday saw the publication of her article. The tiny Post Office, now too long gone but then only yards from our door, kept the *Guardian* for us. It was a half-page spread, and larger than normal. Melanie's sharply serious profile picture stared out at me from the page. An incongruous, but meaningful title, I thought, 'Where the Wild Things Are', a nod to a popular children's book by Maurice Sendak. Written in 1963, it went on to be, and remains, a classic of children's literature. The book forged a fresh new way of connecting to children through their emotions, longings and frustrations. From a review of the book I read, 'Maurice Sendak creates a magical world of imagination, where children can escape to where the wild things are. The heart of the story is that kids have different ways of dealing with frustrations, but they all have one thing in common... they want to be loved unconditionally for who they are.'

I wondered if Melanie had children, and how often she had read this story. I imagined all those *Guardian*-reader parents, affectionately helping their children navigate the world of fearful emotions using these iconic pictures and words. *Was this what Bob was doing back in the prison, back with those 'Lost Boys in Gruesome Land'? Did Melanie see all this, and was the title she chose reflective of it?* Not sure, I continued my quick scan...

Bob was pleased with it. 'It's a clear and accurate account of what I am doing. What do you think?'

'Yes, it's accurate. I wonder what the prison will make of it...'

'Oh, they will be fine, it's good publicity.' And so Bob set off, confident in both his work and the support for it.

Each day John held a morning meeting attended by all the key personnel within the prison, including every wing governor. The meeting was a crucial lubricant for communication, providing an outlet for worrying rumours. It was where John could keep a finger on the pulse of this difficult, closed environment, where he gave out information and received reports. He used it to display his managerial style of firm, enlightened, friendly encouragement, and to push forward his agenda for a culture change: a shift from discipline and control to that of 'dynamic security.' This being the idea that trustworthy relationships are essential for the safety of prisons.

This meeting was held in the board room of the prison. Distant from the wings, it was stuffed with its own importance. Bob always went straight to this early morning meeting before starting work on C-Wing. I wondered if the meeting had read Melanie's article, and what reaction Bob would get, but that morning nothing was said, nothing at all.

The backlash

Bob entered C-Wing to be faced with the most bizarre of unwelcoming committees. Recalling the glass sides of the airlock, and the carefully expressionless scrutiny by officers, it was not to be supposed that Bob's approach could ever have gone unnoticed. I imagined the silent, hostile, but almost gleeful waiting that had preceded his reception.

As the gates slid open, the officer in charge blocked his way: 'You are banned from the wing. You are a discipline and security risk. The men are reacting badly. I can't answer for your safety.' Behind him Bob glimpsed six or seven prisoners walking up the centre of the wing and around the large table at the administrative end, self-consciously carrying placards. Little K had swopped his habitual pint mug of tea for one, just for the occasion. Portly P was grinning somewhat inanely, and B, a large man with flowing locks, was like the others nervously enjoying a spot of rare liberation afforded by the watching officers.

'This is stupid, I will go and talk to them. In no way was the article an attack on them. They can't have read it.'

'No sir, I can't allow that. Remove yourself from the wing.'

'We need to sort this out. I am going to see John, you need to come too.'

'That won't be necessary. Security of the wing is my decision.'

'Yes, it is necessary. It's a serious matter being banned from seeing my patients. It's totally unacceptable. I've driven through blizzards to see them. It's intolerable. You can't keep me from my patients.' Bob replied with a steely outrage which the watching officers had not anticipated. His friendly pleasantness was often mistaken for weakness. And so battle was joined...

With reluctant officiousness, Bob was followed by the peppery little wing governor on the obstacle-strewn route of gates and locks into the administrative block where, in that large office behind that large desk, John was waiting to greet them. He was an experienced Governor, trained in riot control and negotiation, and of course he recognised officer-induced sabotage when he saw it, and clearly knew all about the antics on C-Wing. This was one of his easier adjudications, one for the laughing dinner-table gossip he couldn't resist. But Bob, serious, cut through the hint of patronising amusement: 'I can't be prevented from seeing my patients. They have appointments.' And John, exercising his authority, basking in his role as supreme arbiter of this closed kingdom, declared beneficently, 'Maybe all day is too much, you can go back in the afternoon.'

The wing governor, knowing too the illusory nature of the 'security threat', conceded, grumbling, 'I suppose we can calm them down by then. It's all very well, but it's all more work for my officers. The doctor has to be more careful. These are dangerous men we are dealing with here.'

Back at home I was reading some new European funding proposals, and idly speculating as to whether the morning meeting would be discussing Melanie's article. I thought it showed the prison in a progressive light, and certainly gave a clear account of what Bob was trying to do. And then the phone rang.

'I have been banned from the wing.'

'You've been what?'

'I've been banned from the wing.'

'What do you mean, "banned"? You can't be, it's ridiculous, what's going on?'

'The men were holding placards and walking round.'

'Placards?! What sort of placards, how big were they?'

'They were written in capitals. I didn't take it in at first, but things like DON'T CALL US WILD THINGS and DOCTOR OUT and WE'RE STRIKING.'

'Wasn't anything said in the morning meeting? Didn't you think it was a bit funny? Didn't you pick up any mutterings?'

'No, I just assumed nobody had read it, it was the *Guardian*, after all. Anyway, I was thinking about who I was seeing next. It was a short meeting, not much going on...'

'What are you doing now?'

'It's okay, I'm going back in this afternoon. I'll pick up the bits, and squeeze in the ones I missed this morning. I think I'll give Melanie a ring too, get her reaction.'

'Oh Bob, are you sure?'

'Yes, it's fine, see you this evening.'

His explosive news smashed into my until-then hopeful day. My half-articulated proposal for an education project in Italy suddenly seemed drained of meaning or any urgency. I made myself coffee, it's unreasonable strength now an urgent necessity. Battling through my anxiety, I tried to think. *The prisoners can't even have read it.* I'd never seen a copy of the *Guardian* on the wing. In any case, security screened newspapers and books for items deemed inflammatory or dangerous. Why, I'd even seen copies of *The Friend*, a calmly benign Quaker journal, with names redacted. What was John up to?! He would dignify a barbecue by his presence and support but didn't bother to even visit C-Wing when Bob was being challenged by both prisoners and staff.

True, the Prison Officers Association, the POA, was strong, and John had to tread a careful line between his reforming agenda and their fiercely held practices, and it was only through a combination of jokey charm and persuasive inducements that he was easing in a culture of humanity. So was Bob just an easily-scrapped scapegoat in the almost ritualistic struggle between Governor and governed? An unbidden image of a smirking John came flashing in. I imagined the difficulty he had in keeping a professional rein on his glee at Bob's discomfiture and potential downfall, but it was more than this, more than a head boy triumph.

What was Melanie saying again? What had John expected? What had the officers expected? I read the article again… It was an 'encomium' alright, as Melanie called it, but for Bob, and his work, not for the officers, or their views, or for John. He was only mentioned as giving 'wholehearted backing' to Bob. Melanie had talked to John, talked to the officers, talked to the men, but it was Bob who got the final accolade. 'His work deserves wider scrutiny and application. The implications are enormous, not merely for prison administration, but for the whole spectrum of family and social policy.'

So that was it. They had been ignored, and they were angry. They needed praise too, it was their prison, their prisoners; they were the ones who did the work, kept it together, knew what they were doing, not this jumped-up blathering intellectual of a doctor. How could Bob possibly survive, he wasn't in this team? No matter that his work was beginning to transform lives, as Melanie described, 'from shrunken drugged monosyllables to confident relaxed drug-free articulacy.'

For some, like the dispensing officer behind the Happy Hatch, this was just a further diminishment of their role, of their worth. *What were they for, if these prisoners were no longer dangerous? Wherein lies their status then, their super-special importance?* I remembered the words of that officer on my first visit self-importantly pointing to the slouching line. 'You wouldn't think they were the most dangerous men in the whole prison system…'

Presciently, the article described Bob's theories as a 'challenge to opinion on both left and right': to those on the left who cite poverty, economic and political causes, and those to the right who believe in born-evil criminality. I knew she was right, but I didn't know then just how very isolated a position it was. My natural home was the liberal Enlightenment intelligentsia, from whom I still valued some kind of yearned-for approbation. It was a battle I could see writ large over the prison estate, and the subtext for all the angry scepticism hurled at Bob both from liberals who scorned his emphasis on the individual, and from conservatives who scorned any idea of causation, let alone transformation.

Then I remembered Bob and was scared. It wasn't an intellectual debate for him. They were dangerous men. *What if the connections he's made aren't strong enough? If the officers can manipulate such a charade, they certainly aren't in the business of protecting him, and neither is John.* My now *really* daffy one was deliberately not seeing all this, choosing to ignore it in pursuit of his vision, the cure for violence, and now he was driven by the compact he had made with the men, who against all imaginings had opened their ghastly humiliating fears to him.

I drank some more coffee and stuffed some bread in the toaster. It was a large four-slice affair, brought from our old family home. It had an extra-wide facility for crumpets which accommodated the bread Bob made. However, no amount of toast could stop the sick feeling in my stomach. I was on my own here. I wanted to ring Bob, to shout 'Come home, it's not worth it!' *Oh this is ridiculous, what am I doing, are my worries really real? What if the men weren't play-acting, and really were offended and angry? What happens when you offend a mass of serial killers, hit-men and disordered psychopaths?* Clutching for relief, I wondered if I should ring my sparky friend, but imagining her laughing dismissal I went into the garden instead. She too was caught in a difficult invisible web.

Patches of blue lavender were still hanging on, defying the approaching autumn. Their fragrance was strong as I gently rubbed the stalks between my hands, attempting to blot out the banging images in my head. The waiting garden was still lovely, but now seemed devoid of any allure. The doom-filled cadences of Tennyson's *Morte d'Arthur* crept into my head ... *Comfort thyself: what comfort is in me?* Tennyson too had walked these same coastal paths, gazing out at this ever-moving sea. *What comfort is in me? What comfort indeed!* I was stuck, glued by impenetrable hours I needed, somehow, to clamber my way through.

Now, gazing back at this scene, I am seized with a painful acuity thankfully then unavailable to my still-hopeful younger self. Difficult as it was, frightened as I was by this bullying pantomime, it was just a jokey prelude, merely the first attempt to use the men to destroy Bob. It was standard harassment tactics from a prison officer culture used to seeing off many a threat to their assumed status and power. Neither governors, nor the Prison Service executive were immune from it. John, too, I came to realise, suffered under this burdensome yoke.

An instantly soothing sound hit my ears. 'Sue where are you?' And Bob appeared at the top of the steps. Untangling myself from the shade of an evergreen *magnolia grandiflora,* whose persistent growth, and vast, lemon-scented blooms had offered me a strange comfort, I called out, 'Here! What's going on, are you alright?' I folded myself into his huge hug, a reassuring strength so welcomingly additional to my own. It was instant relief.

'It's fine, I went back in and had some good sessions.'

'What do you mean? What did they say? Why did they do it? What were the officers like?'

'Nobody said anything. I think they seemed a bit sheepish. Anyway, I had a good session with E.'

And so Bob carried on eagerly describing where he was up to. There was more video of E, 'Astonishing stuff! And the man in the blue jumper, well! He wants to have a therapy group with his mates! They're getting there! They just need time now.'

Solidly certain of my interest, he chatted on, but for me, deflated worries collided with an ever-lurking hurt. I released loud heaving sobs. All that swirling agony of waiting, imagining, thinking, identifying, hoping, had been an agony unseen, unnecessary—what had seemed such a pivotal moment, awaiting resolution, my mind chewing and chewing, shaking it all around like a too-excited terrier—all this painful experience, then, only an indulgent second-hand thing, manufactured, not necessary, not useful—essentially meaningless. I was certainly invisible in the beefy drama of the prison world, unnoticed by all those positioned players in the watching arena. *Any visibility I might have is contingent, granted only through a husband's lens: the waiting woman, man back from the wars, what value her agony? What value indeed her waiting? Unbidden, what had I given up for this dangerous madness? Home, job, money, career, and Bob, what had he gained? Nothing but cruel accusations.*

Finding a voice

Looking back, it seems now that it was all an expression of the pain of trying to find my voice in a world where hero narratives are the dominant myth. I was clever, and informed, my feminist consciousness had never really been questioned. It was a part of me, always on alert. I recall schooldays in the fifties, knocking on my fearsome, bullying headmaster's door to tell him the girls wished to watch the final of the local schools' football match rather than be confined to sewing. Patronisingly amused, he'd conceded. It was this consciousness that led me to explore feminist research and therapy, and to early, iconic, angry classics, such as *The Women's Room* and *The Female Eunuch*. Marx, I read, had four daughters who wrote much of his work. This was the hinterland that entwined my exhausted sobbing.

Bob was baffled. 'But you must see how important you are. I couldn't do it without you.'

'I know I know, but I have to feel my value, it has to be real.'

'It is real. How could it not be?'

I had to get back to the meaning. I couldn't find it in words. Words could trap, and render meaning senseless, strangled in a too-tight embrace. I needed my own experience. I thought of the video tapes accumulating in Bob's study, a physical, factual presence. Oblong shapes, carefully coded and dated, they waited in slender metal drawers. *Waiting for what? To give voice to the invisible, to give witness to moments of pain, of clarity, of honesty.* E's words came back to me again. *'I am telling you the truth, aren't I? It's the truth, isn't it... the truth's gotta come out.'*

The videos were undoubtedly real. *They're alive — alive with meaning that requires witnessing. The men need them to be shared, listened to, understood — and so does Bob.* It was a bargain they had with the camera. It wasn't just Bob they were talking to, it was me.

And so, I re-engaged with the project, thinking perhaps that somehow some definitive research, something change-making, could be carved out of all those captured hard won moments. I wasn't aware that this was a radical act, but of course it was. It was giving a voice to the invisible — the invisible that is so easily, so automatically, so destructively unnoticed.

'Did you still manage to video the sessions?'

'Yes, of course.'

'Oh good, so it didn't interfere then.'

'No... but I have to take it further, I have to put it in writing. John needs to know it's not acceptable, barring me from the wing.'

'Yes, but be careful, it's tricky for John too.'

'He can't let the officers behave like that.'

'No, but he probably knows that. Why do you want to send it, will it be worth it?'

'I just need to do it. Even if it's ignored, I will have told him.'

And so, words were sent: carefully crafted memos to Governor John. Into the prison system they flew. Ever multiplying, arriving on desk after desk: wing governor, security governor, chief medical officer, regional office, head office, probation. Destined from the off for deletion, they were shredded into invisibility. How were we to guess that this invisible non-answer would become so potently visible under the lens of the High Court? For now, we only knew Bob was ignored, his words were ignored.

Strangely this episode seemed to usher in a period of calm, a calm I began to rely on. John was amiable and jokey, perhaps satisfied that Bob had been bloodied in the battle: the oh-so-cleverly certain idealist had hit the rocky realities that were the prison system. Bob continued with his quest, his memos now an irrelevance to him and almost forgotten, were tucked well away on the back burner. As for the watching men, this testing spat had revealed something their bruised minds could never have imagined: Bob did indeed trust the truth of what he was saying, and trusted them to engage with him.

This was a time when I felt curiously released, sending a letter to a friend writing that we had reached 'the sunny uplands.' I painted our front door. I loved the light, glass-paned elegance of it; pale lemon would suit it, a colour reminiscent of spring, or summer lemonade, of garden parties and chattering children. Much later it was to revert to a heritage grey-green, reflecting, I suppose, the sombre weight of a more serious time. I was learning to file my fears away, even if not quite demolishing them. My anguish in the garden had shaken and annoyed me. It was too disturbing, too unnecessary, so this became the time to paint my door yellow and reconnect with my old working world, or so I fondly thought.

The Guardian

It was the moment to go to Italy, and to continue something of my own working life. I accepted a request to advise on the development of European-funded courses for women in the deprived Po Valley Delta. I look down at the ageing notebook where I jotted down plans for the trip, and see how I listed what I would wear. Appearance was as significant for the Italians as it was to the Parkhurst officers and the watching men. However, the carefully-gentle unobtrusive garb I wore for my first encounter at Parkhurst would never work there. Puzzling over a note mentioning a 'Green Jacket', I remember an oversize creation with shoulder pads and large lapels, leather ankle boots, high wedge heels and a white cross-cut shirt providing a touch of hopeful elegance and authority.

'Brute' was the worst, dismissive and demeaning adjective for these northern Italians. It meant not merely 'ugly' but carried harsh overtones of an inner ugliness of thought, mind and soul. Inner life was shown outwardly, and outward appearance expressed this.

So off I went back into this clashingly different professional world of meetings with immaculately presented men. Dressed to impress and perfectly groomed, with cuffs, cufflinks, ties, all carefully providing the correct formulaic image, they were charming. Their whiff of aftershave, softly smooth chins and flawless fingernails left me feeling on the unkempt side, and the words! Lengthy streams of rhetoric from all, without recourse to notes: a show of elegant oratory to match the elegance of dress. While all this enjoyable flummery was entertaining me, images of the incarcerated men kept seeping into my vision, an insistent, distracting contradiction to the civility surrounding me, and what of Bob? Back then no mobiles, laptops, or text messages to feed my need for information and reassurance. I had to suppress my anxiety until my return.

The Prison Psychiatrist's Wife

CHAPTER 12

New Man on the Wing

It hadn't, of course, stopped while I was away. Bob, meeting me from the ferry, gave me a huge hug, saying, 'Missed you. How'd it go.' I remembered anew how tall he was. 'Oh okay, got the bones of it. Enjoyed myself. Sorted the report and next stage. What about you? How've you been, what's going on?' Driving home across the fresh green island, the roads winding and quiet, his torrent of eager words taxed my waiting brain.

'Well, we've had an SUSC meeting, and there is a new man on the wing. It's good... he's young, I think he'll make it.'

'A new man? Isn't that difficult? How are the others taking it? Is he a lot younger than them?' I was immediately anxious again. I knew change was destabilising and dangerous: most of the men weren't young, and I'd reassured myself that Bob was managing some sort of settled agreement, and things had been ticking along okay. 'It's fine, it's fine, don't worry.'

But worry I did. Ah, that committee, the Special Unit Selection Committee, tasked with choosing the worst of the worst to send to C-Wing. Unbidden imaginings crept into my mind. Men in suits around a table littered with fat files of reports, protocols and forms. *What emotions were bubbling away, what were they privately thinking, as Bob enthusiastically explained his approach and how this or that ghastly, unstable man could be helped? Would they select someone just too dangerous? Too dangerous to sit alone with Bob... how had they reacted to Bob's memos? Curiosity, disbelief, irritation, anger?* I suddenly remembered the lack of any response.

They were charged with the impossible, making a rational disposition of the irrational. An ever-growing file helped. Selective evidence could be culled from its bowels to be given fresh importance. As a nationally important committee housed in Prison Service headquarters, being useless couldn't ever be questioned. *Let's see how he deals with this one. Hasn't worked in prisons five minutes...*

Bob, unaware of my skittering thoughts, happily chatted on, 'Yes it's going well, I think there's a bit of a breakthrough there... the clue is his real dad.' And then, my silence penetrating as we continued our homeward drive: 'It's okay Sue, it'll be alright, it's a breakthrough. I want you to see it. I'm glad you're home.' I reconnected. 'So am I.' Bob needed to know that I could see what he could see, that I understood, and engaged with, the hard tussle. And well... I too had to know.

Another painful video

The screen filled as a figure turned and positioned himself in the empty chair in front of Bob and the anticipating camera, his back to the cell door. He bent and placed a large mug of what looked, through the murky opacity of white plastic, like tea. I never liked drinking from plastic, it wasn't soothing porcelain like my own favourite mug. Prison issue, I supposed, and the thought followed, *Of course plastic is more difficult to use as a weapon.*

At first this prisoner was a familiar sight. Shoulders hunched to his chest, and arms folded around his body, he seemed slight and shrunken, with an air of pallid ill-health that often hovered over incarcerated men. He was young, too young to be immersed in such bleakness. He rolled his head as if finding bearings in an unfamiliar landscape, and eyes large and dead skittered across dark sunken sockets as Bob cheerfully introduced himself.

'Well now, good to see you H, I'm Dr Bob, let's see... what's the date now?' His gaze is gentle, clear, confident, pen poised over a pad of lined paper, eager to begin the search.

'How old are you now H, and uh... let's see, how long have you been in?' H bends and picks up the mug. It's large, easily a whole pint. Cradling it in front of his face with both hands, emotionless, 'It was my birthday last week.'

'Do you see yourself as having a problem from the past, anything like that?'

'I seen the psychiatrist, he done the tests and says I'm not mentally ill. "I will not recommend you for Rampton, they can't help you there".'

'Do you see yourself as having a violence problem?'

'Yes, yes I do.'

'And you want some help with that?'

'The defence psychiatrist apparently said there is definitely severe personality disorder there.'

'And you agreed with that?'

'Yes, he said, "He is psychopathic, his violence is controlled, it isn't a spur of the moment thing. He had time, it was planned".'

A rehearsed, second-hand, distant chilling answer, a smooth, factual account of a textbook, professional diagnosis. He sounds unconnected, almost bland, indifferent to the enormity of the words. I flinched, and found my hand covering my face protectively, wanting to blot out something... everything.

'Where do you think your violence is coming from?'

'There's been a few things mentioned. The way I am...'

My waiting ears heard a careful, lengthy list of cruelties stretching the length of his young life. This was familiar reportage, but he appeared almost comfortable, unaffected as the dreadful catalogue continued. *How can Bob ever make this better, supportable? It just isn't.*

Then came the question: 'Your real father, what's going on there?'

Suddenly a boyish smile changed his face, the blank blandness disappeared. He appeared young, vulnerable, likeable... *Was it relief?* I couldn't tell. He lent forward eagerly: 'There's hatred there. Deep resentment...' He is animated, emphatic: 'Probably why I am such a bitter person.' And then his face flips back to a cold blandness as he talks about his crime, and how calm he was. I am feeling scared now.

'I admit it, I don't deny what I did. I planned it. I wanted to see what it's like to take a life.' Leaning back in his chair, arms stretched wide, he was a larger figure, more dominant. I noticed attractive, wavy hair, pulled back behind square shoulders, but then it started, a precise, filmic report of the murder, an almost patient description, smoothly rehearsed, factual, and brutal. A brutal, and indeed a most properly objective report, devoid of emotionality and opinion, sticking to the how, the when, the where, spread out in awful detail. On and on and on it went. There was absolutely no clue to the demanding question pounding my brain, grabbing my heart. *Why? Bloody hell, why? All so mightily against sense, reason and humanity. I don't want to hear this.*

A conversation stopper if ever there was one. *What reply was even possible?* He parades his Hannibal Lecter wares before Bob, a cat proud of a bloody catch few could emulate. He stares at Bob. *Did he believe his own account, did he want Bob to? Did I? Did I want to?* Twenty-first century nomenclature for 'born evil' is often described as bad genetics leading to a lack of an empathy centre in the brain. In truth it was a description of what I was now seeing and hearing.

H called it bitterness, a frozen, solid, implacable iceberg of anger, a wound of incalculable hurt. My local shop has a label 'Frozen Promotions.' It fits H's smooth, chilling, promotional oration.

I felt sick. This wasn't some Hannibal Lecter fantasy-fiction, it was actually real.

Then Bob turns to me, 'Look, this is it! He's avoiding the question about his father, I am onto something...' Staggeringly for Bob this chilling response was a clue, hinting at another reality, one that could, perhaps, provide a lever for the transformation that was his quest.

'Stop it Bob! Weren't you scared? This is awful...'

Bob laughs, 'Well I couldn't stop, he was between me and the door!'

Course he was. My bitter thought hit hard...

I wanted to laugh, to be comfortably hysterical. Bob continues, 'But seriously, I had to move on, had to move *him* on... otherwise absolutely no point, no point if all he does is say terrible things, then — then it'll all repeat...'

We looked at each other: the unsaid horror, 'and he might kill again', hung, and floated away...

All this is too absurd, too ridiculous, *The sun's shining for heaven's sake*. I stand up.

'What are we doing sitting here? It's too much, let's go out...' Laughing and cross and mesmerised by the absolute extremity of this situation, I say, 'Oh get me some cake, why haven't we got any bloody cake.' Bizarrely it couldn't be clearer. That was my problem. 'No but there's some biscuits. I'll make some tea.'

Could Bob manage to connect, and find a way of dissolving such bleak anger? Well, he had to try, and I had to more than encourage it, I had to understand, and to look. The only reason to look, the only value it could possibly have, was in transforming this tale of horror. I revived my optimism, and, with both hands around a large hot mug of tea made very weak with an over-abundance of lemon slices, I sat down beside Bob saying, 'Let's start again.'

I watch as Bob persistently, gently continues pressing, pushing, seeking for the person, the feeling behind the concrete facades of explanation. It's a strange sort of dance as trust, the antidote to fear, starts to emerge. Bob calmly, gently questions the words he's given, H tries different ones, testing, testing, seeing if his well-rehearsed bait of explanation will be swallowed.

'Your real father... what's going on there? Have you got over it?'

'Never had the guts to kill myself.' He shuffles, and leaning forward, eyes fixed on Bob, says, 'Have you seen my file?'

'No, I haven't actually, I prefer to hear what you think. What about your real dad... are you angry with him at all, what's going on there?'

Bob pauses, waiting expectantly.

'My psychiatrist... I decided to kill him.'

Bob is answered with a frightening burst of calculating brutal rhetoric. 'I could kill him very quickly... such joy from knowing what I'm doing... people who know me used to flinch and shiver.' On and on he goes...

So that's it then. Feeling mainly relief, I said, 'Bob you can't do this, he's warning you off! Not enough trust to keep going, but enough respect to warn you off.'

'It's okay I touched on something.'

'Touched, touched! Should just about think you did!' I screamed in almost panic. *What on earth is Bob doing, trying to access the poisonous nest of feelings behind the thoughts of this man? I'm seeing the fearful terror of a rejected baby turned into the icy rage of a baby now able to move, to act with fearful intent.*

'It's okay, it's remarkable, he's doing very well. It's only the first time I've seen him. I am two years in now, I know what I'm doing. I can read violence. Just listen to the next bit, we are getting there, you'll see', and moving to turn the camera back on, Bob gives me a hug of encouragement.

But can I? What residual nerves can I summon up to help quell my fears? What understanding, what optimism can I find? I am weary. It's a wonderful ambition, curing violence, but... showing to a fractious world no-one is born evil, that we all emerge sociable and lovable and want to remain so, is a colossal task.

My eyes turn back to that sharply-lit scene. A functional enclosure, a functional chair, nothing to please the eye, not a scrap. Oddly I think, *It can't be smelling fresh, how can anything be fresh, and clean and new? H looks dreadful, how can he not* be *dreadful? Really! What are we thinking?! Isn't it all too much, too not possible?*

A huge sense of loss

Then I hear the words, casual and firm, biting into all the horror with a calm reassurance: 'How do you feel about me saying all this?' Patiently, carefully, Bob is seeing beyond it all ... hearing, listening, with a different kind of sight. H begins to respond ... 'Bitterness, coming from the past ... it's the first time I've said it ... the sooner you can get it out of me the better.'

He was, well ... was he almost confiding? A huge sense of loss seems to drown me in an inexplicable wave of feeling. My mind, my brain, sparks back ... I am looking through hard glass, gazing—clutching at connection with my just-born premature son. He is encased in a plastic box, wired-up to tubes providing all the necessities, it is thought, for his tiny life. I am not allowed to touch him, whisper to him, feed him, stroke him. Indeed, my silent tears are upsetting all the nurses, so an hour a day of gazing was deemed my limit. A few hard weeks later I lift him from his plastic box. He takes as many gulps from my eager waiting breasts as his tiny frame can manage, and sinks into contentment. Trust is returning for him. We take him home. And now so many years later it hits me, this connection to the terrifying howl of an abandoned baby, who might just be learning to trust his adulthood and ask for help.

'Until I come here I knew I'd kill again ... glad I didn't ...'

'You'd rather not?'

'Yes ... now I'm here ... a load off my back.'

'You can see me like this once a week and we'll sort it all out. Thanks.'

A familiar hand, long and shapely, fills the screen offering an invitation. H stands somewhat awkwardly, unused to respect and civility, and surprised he grasps the proffered hand. 'Nice to sort things out like this with you.' Then the screen goes blank. The session's over.

Nice! I laugh and push Bob's knee. 'A bit of an understatement, don't you think?' I am exhausted, we are both relieved; me, because I might be seeing a way through, Bob, because this viewing with me confirms his vision and my support. H had, after all, said it was nice to sort it out like this, so maybe he was becoming less of a danger—and more, I hoped maybe this could be the paradigm breakthrough that really would convince Bob's colleagues ...

CHAPTER 13

Grendon

A brace of ducks arrived on the wing. Shot by the careful principal officer, they were a gift for Bob: a powerful and public statement of support. I wondered fancifully about the lead shot that had been their downfall and whether the security scanner became alarmed.

It was a nice moment. The wing was becoming friendly, less fearful and more purposeful. The officer pack too was reshuffling; a few moved themselves off in muttered disgust, including the irksome dispensing officer, as others requested transfers onto the wing. I got used to our clanging gate bringing optimistic news. We even received an invitation to an officer's wedding.

The ducks were a challenge! Loosely tied together by their skinny necks with some string, Bob carried them into the kitchen. They struck me as quite long and had flappy feet.

'What do you think of these then? T brought them in for me. He's just shot them, shooting is his hobby.' *Of course it would be!* I thought sarcastically, and in truth I was feeling a bit repulsed. The ducks were very dead and a bit grubby. Bob seemed pleased with his present, seeing it as a significant token of acceptance. And I supposed it was a breakthrough for him, but not for the poor oblivious ducks.

'Well, we'll have to deal with them somehow ...'

'I like duck, can't you do it with orange or something?'

'They need to be plucked and gutted before roasting, or you can just try and take the skin off with all the feathers, then we can stew the lot. Might be quicker and tastier, depends how old they are. You have to look out for the lead shot ...'

In the end Bob took them outside, started to pluck them, and then decided on the quicker approach. After simmering them for a while I took out the bones and added mushrooms and onions, straining off not really much fat, whilst thinking *They're lean birds, got quite a lot of flying done in their time.*

We ate them sitting at the table looking down the garden to the sea. I'd never seen ducks here, only occasionally geese flying South in formation, and swallows in early-autumn gathering for their well-rehearsed trip, but always the buzzards circling, hunting... sometimes I saw their flight weighed down by a claw full of struggling rabbit.

Bob interrupted my musings, 'It's really good this stew... it was nice of old T to give them to us. Must take quite a bit of sorting out. I wonder where he goes shooting. You can't do it just anywhere.'

'No', I was wondering that too. 'I saw T that first day I was in...'

'Yes, he would have been there, he basically ran C-Wing.'

A respecter of rank and follower of orders, T rated the importance of his job, and there had been an air about him of careful holding back: any opinion of what John was doing, introducing a clearly maverick psychiatrist into the tightly-controlled world of C-Wing, a world he knew, was deliberately veiled. So the stew tasted extra-nice as we sat and ate together, feeling this acceptance by a colleague for all the hard work we were doing. I realised how very much this was missing, how very much I wanted it for Bob, and then suddenly how much I missed my work, and my colleagues' support. I rubbed my head. It was starting to hurt with an undefined ache...

'Have we any ice cream? I could do with some.'

'Are you alright? What's the matter? Things are going well.'

'Yes, I know they are, it's just it brings it home a bit when someone starts to be nice, it gets through somehow... what we're doing, what we're missing...'

'Yes, but it'll be alright. It's lovely here, isn't it...'

Bob was anxious. He sensed my worry, but he didn't share it. He, after all had the sodding job, I was the onlooker. The thought hit quickly, bitterly, disruptively. I didn't want it. 'Yes, it is lovely... we'll see what happens...'

I allowed myself to think, to feel it was all going to be okay. There was interest, cautious support and hope—*Just another push and it will all calm down*—a hope that was not quite a faithful companion of mine. Tiny ripples, not quite waves of positive connections began to emerge. Bob waved a letter.

Grendon

An invitation

'The Governor of Grendon wants me to talk at their conference. I met him at the Governors' Conference, he wants me to show E. It's great. Do you want to come? I'm sure he'll put you on the list...' I did. I'd read about HMP Grendon. Set up in 1962, it was still termed 'experimental' even after more than thirty years. It managed prisoners with an alternative regime that attempted to mimic a therapeutic community. There were apparently groups run by the prisoners in which their criminal behaviours were remorselessly discussed and challenged. The regime was endlessly evaluated and seemingly the reoffending rate was much less than in standard prisons. It was designed as one of the later stages of pre-release for serious offenders who mastered it.

If Bob's work succeeded and any of the C-Wing men were downgraded from their special status of Category A, the label reserved for dangerous men (and loaded with a peculiarity of meaning within the prison estate: an escape risk, a danger to the public, and for C-Wing men, the extra accolade of 'mad') Grendon was the place they'd likely go to graduate. The criteria for anyone to be sent to this prison were almost the polar opposites of those for C-Wing entry. For starters, they had to volunteer, to want to go and to be motivated to try to change, then to be deemed neither a danger to themselves nor violent, compliant with the therapy and potentially suitable for release. All of which Bob was hoping for his charges.

I was curious. C-Wing Parkhurst was the only prison wing I'd ever entered. I wanted to know what this one would feel like. Maybe an experimental prison could be a gentler berth for Bob. Still stuck with seeing and feeling the enormity and difficulty of what he was attempting, I didn't then—I couldn't—imagine his feral charges ever graduating into this place, after talking about their offences.

We drove to the prison through the soft Buckinghamshire countryside. Bob was animated. 'Looking forward to it, it's a celebration conference. It started thirty years ago. I think all the men will be there, as well as the bigwigs. I wonder what they'll make of E. It's a small prison, only about two hundred.'

I wondered too. Bob intended to give his Governors' Conference presentation. *What bullish egos might be waiting? This time the Prisons Minister would be there, and a mass of careful therapeutic aficionados. The men too would be listening—listening for a wrong beat, a lack of knowledge, empty liberal idealism.*

I shuddered. It didn't do to think too much, I was getting a bit scared. Nervous for Bob, I had a gutting sense that I didn't want to see him on display. It was too hard. He was driving, and legs too long for the car meant a knee was angled toward me. I patted it protectively.

'Bob, be careful. The men ... a lot are lifers, they'll have terrible histories, it might be hard for them to hear you and E. And all the professionals, they have a protective, well-trained certainty.' Bob laughed, 'That's a mouthful! Don't worry, it's not as bad as all that. The men have bullshit meters and recognise reality. The staff, they'll be interested in anything that might take things further. They must be interested. They volunteer to work there. It's unique footage after all.' I knew what he said was right. Using it to squash my fears, I answered, 'Well it absolutely is, you do need to show it, and Grendon ought to be the perfect place.'

We drew up into the car park. An unmistakable prison of unpleasant red brick loomed oppressively large. The security at the gate was familiar, as was the endless lock-unlock regime, but this time there were smiles, acknowledgements and swift progression to the prison hall where men and officers were beginning to cluster. It didn't feel edgy or threatening, in fact it seemed anticipatory and purposeful. I noticed a stage, a screen, and tangled cables. Then the smiling Governor came over and shook hands. To my relief he seemed gentle, thoughtful and interested.

Selecting a seat on the far outside edge of the first row where I thought I might be less obvious, my stomach twanged. It was an environment of total maleness, the hall stuffed with row upon row of intent men. There must have been an occasional watching woman in the ranks of the surrounding officers, the maleness of their uniform masking any lightness, any colour. No-one appeared to notice me, though of course they must have done, and I pushed my chair back, angling it slightly to enable a sideways view of this most unique of audiences. Bizarrely, I was reminded of monks choosing to live enclosed lives of suffering and challenge. *Why all this human misery?* It floated unseen, invisible, seeming to curl around me.

Bob by now was on the stage, busying with the cables and his laptop. It was all too near, too present, too uncomfortable. The audience was starting to settle, to wait. *Anticipating what?* I couldn't tell. Pre-conference nerves I knew of old, but this was something different. I was scared. A dentist-drill scared, a wanting-it-to-be-over scared.

Satisfied, Bob gave a thumbs up to the waiting Governor and looked confidently out over the by now packed audience with a cheery smile. *Of course, he knows what he's doing, of course I am being silly.* My clashing thoughts started to settle.

The gentle Governor was speaking now, welcoming, informing, thanking, introducing. I recognised the role, and the relief that came with the beginning, finally, of any conference. Used to conference arrangements, I could only imagine what level of extra busyness, of detail, security, of double-checking this event had demanded. So over to Bob. The tall figure started:

'We are all born one-hundred-per-cent dependent. If we aren't looked after, we die. The infant knows that. It's the source of extreme terror: I am looking for fear and anger from childhood…'

This wasn't a lecture, it was more than information—the words created a presence and a meaning that hovered over the silent men, clear, confident, both strong and gentle. Bob knew the impact his words could have, and was guiding his audience through the turbulence, inviting trust, a collaboration. Bending, he pressed a switch, and the image of E appeared on the screen, the big man who early on had given Bob his trust. The figure, the cell, the despondency, the air of lifeblood drained, the absence of joy or any glimmer of hope connected viscerally with the waiting men, but as they watched the big man settled, a whiff of almost relief crossing his face:

'It's about me Mum and how she used to batter me as a child.'

Suddenly I was within a room full of an intense peculiarity of listening. Deep expectant stillness surrounded me. It was a sudden recognition, a sudden understanding. These men had heard therapy words many times before, but this was new, the bewildering, discomforting opposite of the words they'd heard before. *These words are fresh and newly minted, and the people who need to hear them, who can authenticate them from within their own lives, are in this room and connecting with them.*

A sense of extreme privilege engulfed me as the uniqueness of this moment sank in. I glanced from the men to the waiting staff, arranged carefully around the edges of the room. *What were they thinking?* I couldn't tell. *Could these words and these images forge new thinking?* Into this listening expectancy crashed a loud, angry voice, hurling a cutting accusation at the calmly explaining figure on the stage. 'You are laughing at him. It's wrong. You should never laugh at a patient. You are wrong. It's not professional.'

The voice was incandescent with determinedly outraged fury. Shocked, turning to look along the front row to the far side, I saw that the voice had a suit and sleek black hair, and more than pointing was throwing his whole arm towards Bob. I learned later he is a forensic psychiatrist. Worried thoughts chased around my brain. *Why, why is this man so bizarrely angry, so out-of-proportion to—what? There was no possible threat... or was there? Maybe to his training, his knowledge, his role, status, and profession—his presence!* I looked around at the expectantly quiet men: this audience was his fiefdom. Was this some playground power battle? Scared, I could almost hear the anger he was inviting: *Making fun of a prisoner? Laughing at him? Who does he think he is?!*

Looking back now this was an ominous, furious portend of the attacks that lay in wait, but back then I felt only relief at Bob's firmly transparent response: 'No, I am laughing with him, it's actually hilarious. It's reality. He's seeing it for the first time. It gets clearer and clearer...'

Bob turned to restart the interrupted video. This time, however, it refused to start. There was a flurry of checking cables, connections, plugs: a growing nightmare, a subdued, waiting muttering. The Governor tried to help, and I noticed the voice had subsided, satisfied, into his chair, arms firmly crossed around him. Suddenly a strong male voice shouted out from the centre of the men: 'You know it all, you know what happens next—don't bother about the film, just tell us!'

So Bob did. 'Thanks for that. I will start again...'

He had a transcript, and of course knew it absolutely. Standing at the front of the stage, he connected directly, explaining the dialogue, the significance: what he looked for, what he heard, what he didn't do, what he found. What the big man said and did, and the thread through all of this, *why?*—what causes such terror, distress and mayhem. The prisoner was right. He could and did just tell them. It was powerful, engrossing and truthful. More than compassion, and more than understanding was on display. Bob was offering a solution. This must have connected to the professional looking man seated behind the table to one side of the stage, for as Bob closed the presentation, he leapt up and striding forward shouted 'Eureka!' and shook Bob's hand. He was later introduced to me as the medical director of the prison.

We join a therapy group

Men and staff were standing now and slowly, almost reluctantly I thought, moving through the doors back to their wings. I made my way somewhat cautiously over to Bob's little group of chatting staff. I noticed the kindly-looking man who'd stood up at the end and thanked everyone for their efforts, saying how pleased he was to be here, how important Grendon was, and how impressive the rehabilitation figures. I later learned he was the Minister for Prisons. Bob seeing me, turned and said, 'The Governor says we're invited to visit a group on the wing, are you up for it?'

'Yes, love to … are you sure I'm invited?'

I knew that invitations to the groups were at the discretion of the whole group itself. This was a fixed rule, and part of the therapy process at Grendon aimed at fostering responsibility, independence and self-control. 'Yes you are. We can have a cup of tea there …' I recognised Bob's mood, he was delightedly chatting, ebullient and animated, pulling all along with his enthusiasm and optimism. It had been a triumph. His message and his ideas, his understanding, had indeed connected, but for me, somehow lurking around, were my not-quite-doubts. I couldn't ignore such a disturbing anger, or indeed that we were actually in a Category B prison, where many of the men were sex offenders. Uncomfortably, I was both pleased and trepidatious. Not in control of events, my thoughts were shouting, *Calm down, just stop for a bit! Let's look, let's ask questions — let's see what the prisoners think!*

An officer was on hand to escort us through the prison to where the waiting men were gathered. It was cleaner, fresher than Parkhurst, not so many internal gates, and so far a welcome absence of menace. Grendon was indeed much smaller than Parkhurst, and all the men had volunteered to be there, and I supposed so had the staff, but it was still a prison, stuffed with men, with memories, with misery, despite its overall attempt at understanding. I felt an urge to grab Bob's hand to signal encouragement, some 'well done' solidarity.

In truth, I was gasping for a loving touch. Instead, I walked quietly beside him, only interrupting the chat to ask how many men were in the group.

'There will be about ten, maybe more, and of course they can leave, if they want to...' This normally unremarkable fact was a huge yielding-up of control within the prison system. The officer was conscious of this. I couldn't tell whether he approved. In any event, he didn't want to comment further. We soon reached our destination. Unlike Parkhurst there was an attempt to make the place nice. Low-level padded leatherette chairs were ranged in a circle around the room. Although armless, they were comfortably wide. And so followed the strangest of seminars—and of introductions:

'Hello, I am Bob's wife, thanks for allowing me to come... I like to see what he gets up to!' I smiled a bit, and looked around the circle, where I connected to some reassuring, welcoming nods. The circle too seemed relieved I was there. It's only now, as I gaze back at that strange meeting, I see that I was a protective bodyguard—not for Bob, but for the men. I diluted Bob. I rendered him more normal, more accessible.

Bob plunged in. 'So... it's good to be here, to see you all, thanks—what do you do here? Does it help?' I recognised his gentle, interested probing. The group responded. They were eager, proud of their achievements in surviving this all-challenging regime. *They describe the purpose with a brutal clarity, almost, verging on the masochistic, tinged with bullying.* I quickly squashed the thought. Whatever else, this was a vigorous attempt to engage in rehabilitation. *Here, they tell us, they have to own up to what they have done, to confront themselves, and tell each other the reality of their actions, their emotions, their victims, the harm, their offending behaviour. Here there are no excuses and no hiding place.*

Some men were louder than others, stronger, larger, more definite, but even those slighter and more fearful appeared to agree. More men were crowding into the room now. All seemed focused on gaining Bob's approval. They knew how horrible they were, what they'd done, and the harm they'd caused. They knew it all in absolute gruesome detail. They were learning how they might control their 'triggers': thoughts, events and actions that could inflame their ever-lurking nastiness.

How could they live with these constant, dreadful reiterations? What kind of knife-edge were they living on, the constant anxiety in their thoughts? I wondered too how hearing the gruesome actions of others reinforced what they thought of themselves; and the staff, *How did they manage this remorseless diet?* Traumatisation by proxy was a new thought back then.

Bob was talking now, 'Well what did you think of my talk? I am a contradiction in terms, a happy psychiatrist...' The questions came fast, and more than interested, they were desperate to know if there really was hope, a further pathway beyond their present experience. Bob's responses were clear, confident and definite. Not second-hand, or repetitious, they were authentic: wrought from hard experience of what he'd witnessed. 'Yes, there are reasons. Yes, terror can be dissolved. Yes. Change is possible.'

It was the most intensive seminar I'd ever experienced. No question of any fidgeting at the back. The men's very survival, their essence, were engaged in the questioning. That Bob was kind and well-meaning was not in doubt, but the men had met that before. I suddenly saw that his was a kindness tempered to a steely utility in the flames of a dreadful understanding. This was what the men were connecting to. This was what they were starting to trust. It was an understanding I found hard and painful. Feeling shaky I shifted in my seat, the leatherette seeming a bit sticky by now, and reached for the mug I'd placed on the floor. I wanted to leave.

Driving back in the car in the early evening we chatted, digesting, developing the day. 'The Governor wants me to run group sessions there... that was the medical director who shouted "Eureka", he's keen.' I thought of the men. Like the man in the blue jumper, they dragged at something in me... but this time it seemed clearer. They were stuck in what awful knowledge they had, in a dreadful remorse, fearful of repeating their actions. They knew the how, and what of what they'd done, but not the why. Their so-far-unknowing unknowable intent.

'That's encouraging, didn't realise he was the medical director, but what about that man at the front? That was a bit over-the-top... who is he?' 'Oh, they said he's a forensic psychiatrist, a bit stuck in his ways, nothing to worry about.' I felt myself trying to be satisfied. If they were fine with it, so should I be. I allowed myself to feel excited, almost happy. It was, after all, the perfect training ground for Bob's approach. This was where it could spread, be evaluated, researched and adopted elsewhere. I even achingly reflected on using my own skills...

'I think it's wonderful, more than could be expected. Well done, you need to spread out from Parkhurst, this is the perfect opportunity.' 'Yes it is...' Bob was excited too. 'I can still work at C-Wing... I couldn't possibly stop. The men at Grendon, they're already on the way, used to groups after all. I can really use what I've learnt.'

Signs of progress

Maybe this was going to be it, we thought, chatting happily into the evening back home in our calm island newness — the time when the challenge, the hard work, could be transferred to mainstream thinking, into mainstream practice. Suddenly yearning for some certainty, I went outside, stood and listened to the distant sea. It seemed louder at night. It knew where it was going alright. Noticing a quickly swooping bat, I shouted for Bob to come and see. I was exhausted. We sat on the old garden bench from up North, already covered in fronds of grey-green lichen, a tribute to its newly relished clear air. Maybe, just maybe, it was all going to be all right.

And it was true, there were the beginnings of much interest in what Bob was attempting. Reforming groups and organizations were beginning to get in touch. Bob's monthly *Guardian* column 'In the Prison Psychiatrist's Chair' was getting noticed. Had John really picked up on a freshly-liberal *zeitgeist* when he tempted Bob down two years ago? I thought of John's sharp awareness, and his eyes constantly on the move, taking in the messages that were there to be had, sifting, weighing, and balancing their importance. It was comforting to think so. My longed for hope started to grow, watered by enthusiastic reports from a Bob revelling in the joy of experiencing his work beginning to succeed, and the men starting to blossom.

Practical solid signs too began to emerge. 'B wants to make you a table in the workshop, wants to know what style you'd like.' B, one of the most frightening men on C-wing, one of the demonstrators against Bob after Melanie Phillips' article in the *Guardian*, was a large man with tied-back hair and a solid, detached, watching presence. At the barbecue I had felt a distant menace, but now sensed only tears as those casually normal words hit my ever-alert brain with a sudden, wrenching sensitivity of feeling. Sniffing and searching for a tissue, elusive as ever, I rubbed my eyes. 'Oh Bob...'

'What's the matter, you funny old thing... it's good news, he just wants to make you a table. It's just that... it's what he doesn't want to do, he just wants to be nice.' Strangely it was the absence of threat that unravelled my feelings. *He didn't want to kill Bob. He didn't want to be nasty. He actually wanted to make me a table, to be normal, to be liked, to create something for my approval. I was to be the recipient of a carpentry project.* It had unnerving echoes of school, and the proudly presented work of my own children. It was both lovely and heartbreaking. I still have the table. I had requested a small, round one, pedestal-style, and it's used for the telephone now. One of its three, small, curved legs came out of the joint on the main pedestal, and bits of excess white glue are visible from Bob's none-too-neat but efficient repair job. I mean to scrape them off sometime, and possibly paint it a summery chalky white, but for now it still has its layers of shiny varnish, covering the cheapest of wood from a prison workshop.

And then there was P. I had flinched from his intrusion at the barbecue, and he had repulsed Bob's attempts at engagement. However... 'Guess what. P listened to the interview I gave on Radio Solent.' I had listened too. It was powerful, straightforward, and very clear. Bob had described the work he was doing at Parkhurst, the challenges presented by the men, their problems, and his certainty about transformation. The interviewer had been questioning and interested. There was clearly an importance attached to Bob, and the work he was doing.

'Yes, and he came up to me and said, "That was me you were talking about, wasn't it?"'

'And were you?'

'I was talking about how the men have zero self-esteem, and that there was a man who wouldn't talk to me because I'd said I *didn't* think he was rubbish but he himself did.'

'So then what?'

'So he's talking to me now. It's curious... got an extra dose of valuing from my talking about him on the radio.'

'Well, amazing... maybe he got extra reassurance somehow from the public importance of it.'

'Maybe... anyway, we are getting stuck in...'

So began our fun times. As the intensity of my protective energy subsided, so Bob's energies exploded. His monthly column for the *Guardian* started to attract much interest: 'Your *lair*' I sometimes teasingly called it, but it was more than teasing, it was a demonstration of relief, a beginning of normality, a bit of trust that life was starting to become unthreatening, and I could relax and enjoy myself.

Word spreads…

Practically there was much for me to do. As requests and enquiries grew, a second telephone line was installed in my study, along with a fax and answering machine. Radio and TV reporters were the most insistent, often intrusive in repeating requests for interviews and comments. I became used to winnowing out the chancers and the demanding ill-paid researchers from the serious. Journalists were often more interesting, more cleverly nuanced in descriptions of their investigations, and how they wanted Bob's insights! We kept an A4 day per page diary for details and my scribbled comments.

So now 'What's been going on?' became the more usual refrain as Bob entered the kitchen. I bought a cream concertina file to keep track of the documentation for his pending engagements, and a large year planner for the wall to block out the times. All very necessary, I thought, for organizing, avoiding clashes, and prioritising events. I was busy, and happily optimistic. How could I have known that my carefully constructed concertina file was to be used for a bizarre, and vitally different purpose, in the hands of a High Court barrister?

No, this was a time when Bob felt, we both felt, there was an opportunity to influence and change the gloomy, not to say nihilistic, perceptions about what it was possible to achieve with severe personality disorders, and so Bob responded with writings, presentations, workshops, interviews, discussions, and radio and TV appearances. He was intent on showing and discussing the transformative impact of powerful human conversation through his dialogues and films with men who had killed, but it was perilous stuff helping the horrible with a belief in rehabilitation and transformation. He was treading on volcanoes of hurt and anger whenever he was invited to talk in public. He didn't flinch of course:

'It's the only way through, understanding it. Revenge can't help, it hurts everyone.'

'I know, but be careful', I said, flicking a bit of fluff from his jacket before taking my seat in the television studio. Bob was on a panel with an articulate right-wing journalist and a woman whose son had been murdered. Her anguish was painful to see and to hear. And so it started: the modulated tones of the journalist—accusatory, damning and coldly angry.

'You are respecting murderers more than victims, and this poor woman...you are a waste of tax-payers' money, you shouldn't be doing it. They don't deserve help.'

The audience clapped. Oh, this was horrible, Bob was going to be publicly slaughtered. I knew all these popular sentiments of course, but avoided reading them, hoping they wouldn't entangle us too much. Having this mother here was just awful, how could it help her? My face began tingling with little sparks of pain. Covering the cheeks with my hand, I felt the heat. Bob, sitting beside the anguished mother, turned and addressed her directly, 'No, that's not it, the only possible reason for doing what I do is to prevent it ever, ever again, that this dreadful, awful thing won't happen to anyone else. I am not excusing anything, or anyone, I am trying to find out how we can stop it.'

I saw the compassion, his kindness, the desire to help, his strength, and hoped she did too, but how could anyone ever recover from such a thing? A glimpse of our precious son flooded in unbearably. She seemed to connect a little, saying something like 'Well I don't know...'

The journalist wasn't about to be won over however: 'That's liberal nonsense, ridiculous, we all know how to stop it—lock them up and throw away the key. That's what prison's for, to stop it, to punish, to set an example. Decent people won't stand for it.' A ripple of assent moved through the audience.

'I'm afraid it doesn't stop it. Sadly some of the men I treat have killed while in prison. The thing we must do is to focus on prevention, finding and stopping the causes.'

It wasn't to be the bloodbath of my imaginings, and there was a degree of respect for Bob, if not his position. Maybe some seeds were sown. I was imagining, too, the peculiar anguish of all those mothers whose sons had murdered others. Where could they seek compassion and any understanding? I began to follow the politics of crime and punishment. A new Home Secretary, declaring 'prison works', promised to condemn more and to understand less. Setting a new tone, he began reviewing sentences. Naïve and inexperienced, still crammed with an optimism now fed by increasing amounts of goodwill, my interest was one of curiosity, not foreboding. However, this harsh change of culture was to have consequences far beyond my imaginings—consequences that even then were beginning to unfold...

Many intertwined, carefully balanced understandings between governed and governing, between Home Office and Prison Service, prison officers and prisoners, civil servants and the Home Office, were beginning to crumble, as the onslaught of populist political dictums impacted. They were winding their way, Medusa-like, through the gargantuan complexities of the Criminal Justice System, still to surface near us.

Maybe the bad news from Grendon was part of this, we never knew. Ringing Bob, an embarrassed medical director had said, opaquely, 'You are welcome to visit but you can't see the men.'

CHAPTER 14

Prison Politics

A visit to the Home Office

Lunch with Bob brought good news. 'I met the Prisons Minister today, Peter Lloyd. He was very interested in what I'm doing, and he invited me to London to talk about it. I want you to come with me.' 'Are you sure that's allowed?' 'Of course, I'll get a pass for you too. We fix it all up with his office.' Allowed or not, it wasn't usual. I wondered what John thought. 'Oh, John invited me to meet him, Lloyd wanted to talk about C-Wing. John heard Lloyd invite me to London. It's exciting, he's a nice man, clearly into rehabilitation and knows a lot about prisons.'

The Home Office building wasn't one of those proudly placed edifices, monuments to empire, that grace much of Whitehall. This was a modern, ugly, functional building which had grasped its space from a street that must once have housed middle-class Edwardians. I stared at the blank blinds of the glass frontage. It was just over the river from Waterloo station, a convenient if unlovely spot, and not far from Prison Service headquarters. It was here the Prisons Minister had his office. Bob was right, he was a nice man, and clearly committed to his work, which he saw as making the prisons safer and more humane, finding ways to reduce crime and recidivism. His office wasn't as large as John's, the desk not as vast, but a sense of power and purposeful authority pervaded his questioning. Bob was his usual passionate, optimistic self, and as I scribbled his comments in my notebook I was loving it. Here was someone who rated the endeavour, and had the authority to take it forwards.

'I need evidence, facts', he said so that he could do this.

'I'm taping the therapy, they are clearly changing, the results can be analysed.'

'I need a short paper, some outcome indicators.' I butted in, 'How about absence of alarm bells and a massive reduction in medication?' 'That's the sort of thing ... get it to me as soon as you can.'

Looking back now I wonder what the Minister thought. *Was he merely indulging a hopelessly idealistic couple, or was he too hoping for change? He must have been aware of the threat to liberal penal policy. In any event, maybe it was a welcome interlude of optimism in what must be a remorselessly gloomy in tray of problems.*

We'd all managed to joke a bit. Whatever, it thrust Bob into a burst of happy energetic activity, as he tried to gather statistics for a paper that could provide evidence of positive change. In such a bureaucratic institution, there were mountains of records and statistics, all jealously guarded by protocols of almost paranoid proportions. He never did get access to staff absences, which we thought would be a strong indicator of reduction in work stress, consequent on the men being less dangerous, but he did produce a paper with graphs, statistics and conclusions that documented a ninety-five per-cent reduction in medication, alongside a falling to zero of violent incidents and alarm bells rung. It flew from a satisfied Bob onto many a desk.

The attack

Settling into a calmer sense of welcome normality, my high-alert sensors were having a bit of a rest and I was fiddling about with something when I heard Bob come in. Instead of the usual cheery greeting there was, 'Don't worry it's okay.' Alarmed I turned and saw Bob, still in his grey anorak but with a huge swelling lump around the left side of his mouth. The lip had suffered most, I saw bits of blood.

'Bob whatever's happened, you look awful ... sit down.' 'It's alright, it's nothing ... I was a bit silly, misjudged things and S ... he hit me.' I remembered S, he'd been at the barbecue. He seemed so young, so harmless, a pretty little boy.

'I didn't know they'd moved him to a hospital cell from C-Wing, they should've talked to me. I'd had some good chats with him on C-Wing, I was picking up on that. It was my fault, I didn't clock he was actively hallucinating ... I should have waited a bit before charging in.'

'Oh Bob, you have to look after yourself. Let me look at it. Do you want a cup of tea, or is it too sore?' 'It's so clear... fear was driving his hallucinations, the only way he could stop me was by lashing out.'

This of course was the cliff-edge on which Bob was always teetering, chancing his safety against his skill. Battered with a mountain of feelings, and fearful of an emotional unravelling, I'd only been able to offer the simplest of responses. Bob was satisfied he knew why it had happened, and how to stop it. He would talk about it at the next morning meeting. And no, he didn't want to press charges, this was his mistake. The officers were concerned and supportive, had offered tea. Bob was impressed by their unusual understanding. I suppose briefly Bob was one of their own, a comrade wounded in the battle that defined them, though one was heard to mutter, 'That's it then, he'll be off sick, that's the last we'll see of him for a bit, at least three weeks. Doc's made a mess of this one!'

Reported at the next day's morning meeting when Bob appeared as usual, this was the focus of relieved and welcome hilarity as the sceptical officer himself was revealed to be off sick. It was a moment of support, of respect. I allowed myself to think of it as a bit of a breakthrough. Bob was pleased, but as ever, his attention was on the work, and how best to re-engage with S, to get him back to C-Wing. I only knew I wanted to protect Bob. I also knew I couldn't. Talk about a goldfish bowl!

I imagined Bob, walking down the airless, graceless wing, the watching officers so carefully-correct and noncommittal and the men lurking, aware, nothing to do but think, notice and react. Even the piranha was watching, circling, waiting for the next poor guppy. This was the day job alright, needing grit, determination and optimism.

Sadly, this was the last time Bob was to see S: managing dangerousness was the prison's delight, and S was sent on his not-so-merry way. I was to see him once more, however.

A new Director-General of Prisons

Fresh from managing the complexities of a media empire, and a believer in 'walking the floor', Derek Lewis, the new HM Prison Service Director-General, came to visit Parkhurst. Apparently, he even visited the man in the cage.

Bob met Lewis in John's office. He was the supremo, and now accountable for the running of one-hundred-and-thirty prisons. I wondered how he liked his latest empire.

'What was he like? Was he interested?'

'Well, I pointed to the statement on the wall about prisons being places of rehabilitation. He was a bit noncommittal.'

'Oh Bob, he's a civil servant, of course he's careful about what he says, but did he listen?'

'Yes, I talked about what I was doing and its success, and how it needs evaluating and spreading. And he agreed.' 'Well then you silly old thing, that's good news. I expect the Prisons Minister had been talking to him.'

I was proved delightedly right when a memo from Derek Lewis himself requested the Prison Service Research Department to evaluate Bob's work, 'using some of the outcome indicators I have discussed with Dr Johnson.' Unusually, it mentioned meeting Bob, Bob's impressive results and 'infectious enthusiasm.' Lewis wanted it done quickly.

As we pottered about the kitchen, eventually making an evening meal, I was a little lightheaded. A snatch of carefree song came waltzing in, *I could have danced all night*... It was all a bit unfamiliar, this carefree sense, this absence of—what? Of feeling beleaguered. I hugged Bob.

'It's great. The Prisons Minister and the Director-General are behind it. You are being taken seriously... all it needs is a serious look. You can train others, it can be developed.'

This time of approval and the beginnings of support gave me an entrancing glimpse of a future where violent, nasty behaviour could be understood and changed, where the roots of it start to be eliminated and policy changes... my mind rushed ahead... *Implications not only for penal policy but health and education too...*

Corridors of power

My optimism seemed to be confirmed when Bob was invited to address a Select Committee in the House of Lords. We had put together a position paper in collaboration with the National Association for the Care and Resettlement of

Offenders. It was received with interest, and times and a date were allocated. Bob had decided to invite N, a former prisoner, who could add his voice and, Bob thought, extra weight and authenticity to his presentation. So now we were on the early morning train to London, and I was checking through the arrangements.

'What's the procedure for getting in? What entrance do we use, have you got the passes? Are you sure about N's pass?' N had been referred to Bob by a benign GP who'd recognised his adjustment problems. Delighted with his progress, Bob had invited him to tell the Select Committee of his experience. He'd enthusiastically agreed. 'Yes, it's all fine, I've got them all here. N is going to meet us outside at the St Stephen's entrance before we go in.'

In a bit of a mother-hen overload I chattered on, 'Oh dear, I think maybe he should've come with us on the train, does he know his way round London? It's a bit different from the Isle of Wight, he's probably nervous, do you think he'll turn up?' 'Stop fretting Sue, he'll be there. It's going to be fun.' And there he was, waiting on the pavement outside the Houses of Parliament. He was a big man, younger than me with muscly arms. It must have been a warmish day as I could see his large tattoos wending their way up bared arms to disappear under the sleeves of a t-shirt. He was grinning delightedly.

'Hi N, good to see you', said Bob, 'You got here okay then. This is my wife Sue, she's coming in with us too.' 'Yes, no problem … nice to meet you Sue.' 'And you', I said, shaking his hand. I meant it. What committed support he was demonstrating! Listening to them talk together, I hardly knew what I had been anticipating but it wasn't this. *It wasn't this amount of confidence, this eagerness to tell his story, to have his voice heard. Maybe this would make the telling difference, and provide the evidence to convince the policymakers.*

We approached the hugely ornate building, built years after Parkhurst at the height of Empire, but for a not-too-dissimilar purpose, a demonstration of State power. Parkhurst power diminished the powerless: it was, after all, built to house those most dangerous of creatures, young boys, before their transportation to the colonies; Westminster power was built to house elite male privilege — to magnify the powerful.

A frisson flashed into my head, the tiny tickle of excitement I'd had when, as a young political activist, I'd walked through these corridors and first sensed the privilege, the power that could make things happen. It had been a seductive, alluring bubble, until I talked to a fresh new Member of Parliament. There was apparently somewhere to hang his sword, but no office. Waiting in the queue for the all-too-familiar security, I wondered what I'd feel this time. Well, they were corridors of power alright, quiet corridors sheltering a hidden, enclosing power of exclusivity: hail the hallowed walls, curling around us like a fog. How could we ever get through it? Bob of course was charging on, talking animatedly to the official showing us to the committee room. I sensed the odd backward glance at N, whose absence of suit had placed him firmly in the 'workman' (or worse) category.

The committee room had tall, ornate, polished, wooden doors, reflecting a hidden army of cleaners I supposed, as well as the supreme importance of what happened within. They fitted Bob's height alright, unlike the boy-height of his clanging metal Parkhurst office door. The Select Committee was waiting when we entered, ranged along important tables facing us, their agenda and questions carefully placed. The room had a whiff of the courthouse. All be-suited, they were groomed in a necessary unison reflective of their shiny power. Whatever they were anticipating it wasn't us. They were shocked. *Whoever had allowed a man without a suit, a large man with bulging muscles, a man with tattoos, short haircut, and jeans, into this room of dignity and privilege? A man, what's more, who was introduced as a former prisoner.* They were more than shocked, they were frightened. They didn't want to listen. When N stood up to talk, they cut him off: 'Thank you we have the information we need.' They were blithely engaged in making policy and had never encountered any of the men it concerned, and it seemed either didn't want or see the need to.

Outside once through the seal of security, I heard myself breathing great gulps of fresh free air.

'It's nice to be out of that place.'

'Yes. What did you make of it N? Thanks for coming. You made an impact.'

'Well, they didn't seem that interested or know much. Interesting to see inside though...' N was still cheerful. He'd come along to help Bob. He knew how his life had been transformed. What they did didn't matter to him. He was on track.

Back on the train, I was cross, intemperate and tired. 'Wow, I didn't expect that. I thought they might be sceptical, but to not even listen! What was the point? When do they ever take off the blinkers?! Were they born with them, born with silver bloody blinkers not even sodding spoons?!' It'd been a long day, and I was disappointed. I realised just how unreasonably hopeful I had allowed myself to be.

Bob laughed. 'N seemed fine with it though.'

'Yes, it was great of him to come.'

'But they were frightened to see reality, to see that the very purpose of their committee was sitting in front of them, how do we get over that one?' 'It's okay Sue, the results will speak for themselves. Everyone wants prisons to be safer and men less violent.'

It was late, the train was empty. As we rattled along, I felt a little chilly and snuggled up to Bob saying, 'That's true', and indeed it was, but tugging at my mind was whether that could ever be enough. I wanted to be cheerful, after all what we were offering was hugely beneficial. Resting back on Bob's reassuring certainty, I allowed myself some sleepy calm, whilst Bob, taking advantage of the empty carriage, stretched out long legs, his stockinged feet on the seat opposite. Never one to be bored, he was reading a carefully folded article plucked from his breast pocket for just such an occasion...

An outside view

Bob and I often had lunch together in the Arts Centre which was housed in a crumbling eighteenth-century warehouse on the quayside in Newport harbour, only a mile or so from the prison. Our lunches began to take on more of the flavour of a seminar as journalists and media people seeking stories, reformers seeking solutions, and families seeking help pounded Bob with questions, ideas, enquiries and requests.

One of these was Nick Davies, a freelance investigative reporter working on a piece for the *Guardian*. I'd read some of his work and considered it responsible and socially aware. He specialised in lengthy in-depth articles with a narrative rather than polemical approach. Lunch was of course not the purpose of his visit, so coffee cup, notebook and pen to hand, he listened, listened and wrote. Bob, never one to miss lunch, ate the specialty thick vegetable soup with bits of macaroni and talked and talked.

Nick was a quietly strong-looking man, sober and serious. As Bob chatted on, I sensed a growing interest in an unusual story. Bob of course was talking about the work, its importance, its success, how it needed to be transferred, if it worked in Parkhurst with *these men* it would work anywhere. The journalist was more interested, I thought, in Bob and his story, not so much the ideas. A whiff of professional irritation appeared to emerge when Bob discussed his own *Guardian* articles. This was clearly a man confident in his craft, and top of the investigative tree. I wondered afterwards what he'd craft out of Bob's barrage of talk. Unlike with Melanie Phillips, I couldn't tell what he was thinking.

Armed with Bob's thoughts, off they went into the prison, Nick to an interview with Governor John, followed by a visit to C-Wing and the men, Bob to his appointments list. There had been a formal request from the *Guardian* and John, rightly proud of his governance in C-Wing of the most dangerous men in the system, had willingly agreed. It was an opportunity to showcase Parkhurst and his innovative liberal ideas. *He rather enjoys publicity,* I thought, remembering the framed newspaper cartoons on the walls of his loo at home, and his chuckling dismissal of these more-than-obvious attacks. He'd become a favourite target of *The Sun*, with snippets of gossip fuelled by more punitively-inclined officers, but this was a bit different. This was a serious newspaper, a serious reporter, given pages to write a serious story. I now know John must have cleared it further up the line with the press office and regional director. The prison system was ever careful as to how it presented itself.

Back home I started to fret. It's all very well Bob wanting to get his ideas out there, but how can we be sure it won't lead to unforeseen harm, like Melanie's article did? *I'm not sure I like publicity...* It was head-hurting stuff, and of course I was powerless. 'How did it all go do you think, did he get it? What was John like? Did Nick talk to the men?' 'He saw John, and came on the wing. Talked to some of the men. I wasn't there, but I think it went okay, he seemed to understand. We'll have to see what he writes.'

The tiny Post Office and newsagent only yards from our home always kept the *Guardian* for us back then. It was a pleasant ritual, strolling to collect it, having a bit of a chat with the cheery woman behind the counter, then reading and dissecting it over a coffee. Saturday's larger edition we especially enjoyed. The next weekend a commanding four pages were spread across the weekend section of the paper, complete with pictures. Skim-reading it, I saw it hadn't showcased Parkhurst, and didn't mention John. It challenged the Home Secretary, showed Bob as a lone pioneer, 'a natural rebel', whose work sought to demonstrate that what the Home Office was doing was absolutely wrong, and, by implication, ditto John and the prison officers. On the face of it a gripping story, a journalist's dream I suppose. *Against the odds our hero is courageously surviving all manner of perils to forge a new world of reform.* It was a narrative, easy, compelling and an interesting read. So interesting that I was later to meet up with a film director who pulled it out of her handbag declaring she'd kept it for years, wanting to pursue it. There was no doubt it was a positive story, and liberal reformers would be encouraged by it.

Political rhetoric was now beginning to turn vehemently against those in favour of prison reform. 'If you can't do the time, don't do the crime', a catchy blasé mantra along with 'understand less, punish more.' My stomach hurt. I hated reading our dedicated life journey spread out in an almost clichéd logic. I couldn't read it as a liberal reformer, delighted to see an article supporting my views. No, this was Bob, us, me. He'd described Bob physically as 'like a stork in a suit', but that wasn't it. It seemed to read like a favourable school report from a punctiliously objective teacher; including the men's fearful stories it was accurate and true and I found it disturbing. *Guardian* readers were a rarity on the island, and unusually I was thankful. *Was this all really too much daylight for the prison?*

'What's a bloody "natural rebel"?' I growled. 'Nobody's born a rebel. You chose to follow your thinking, to follow the truth of what you've learnt.'

'Shush Sue, it's alright, a bit journalistic, but he's got the gist of it, the roots of criminal behaviour. Maybe people will listen. He talked to the prisoners after all.'

'I don't like him calling you a stork.' But that really was the least of it, and I see now how it was always going to be so much more than an interesting story in a liberal-minded newspaper. The onset of Michael Howard as Home Secretary had meant a change of ethos, and with it the evaporation of political support for liberal ideas about prisons. Peter Lloyd would soon be gone. It served to hasten the encircling forces of anger, and cynicism, forces I was glimpsing with a hard discomfort. Bob couldn't share these glimpses with me as his extreme focus took over: the article shone a national, searching spotlight into Parkhurst, and Bob's work was removed from a tolerated, eccentric obscurity, and became the object of public complaint.

John had overtly to distance himself, support his officers and justify his actions in appointing Bob. It was only later I came to realise, and in the cruellest of circumstances, just how impossible his job had become. He was bounced between the loudly conflicting demands of a powerfully raucous Prison Officers' Association, Home Office civil servants, newly-minted political mantras, and the ever-present tabloid press. The response was swift, a long letter from John to the *Guardian* extolling the work of his officers and condemning the 'lone hero' narrative of the article. Bob sent a short memo to the staff on C-Wing, regretting its tone. He continued determinedly, still talking, still filming, building up his archive, his certainty, his understanding, but what damage was done! Alarmed by the unpleasant incident, I saw how fragile were Bob's footprints in the shifting sands of prison-system politics.

CHAPTER 15

Murder Threat

The telephone rang. By now I had defended myself with a second line, and the phone waiting on the table my side of the bed was reserved for family, close friends, and extreme emergencies. My worry sensors twitched as the faces of our children flashed into my disturbed sleepiness.

'Sue speaking.'

'Is that Mrs Johnson?'

'Yes.'

'This is a C-Wing officer. I shouldn't be telling you this, but could you tell Dr Bob to watch his back? H has threatened to kill him tomorrow.'

It had been a long night. I'd prowled around sipping hot milk, nutmeg and honey, then gone outside, gazed around in the darkness and heard the crashing sea below, its sound magnified in the still night air. Bob was again sleeping soundly as I slipped, as gently as possible, back into our bed. I needed the reassurance of his sleeping presence. *No doubt in the morning he'll call me a silly old thing and say I was overreacting.* I hoped I was.

A puzzle to solve

Breakfast time saw Bob slicing his bread and stirring his porridge. Bread was a peculiar specialty of his. He purchased sacks of wheat grains, which he then ground into flour. The resulting bread was fresh, dark, and dense with a strong nutty flavour.

'Bob I am worried. I don't know what's going on.'

'It's a bit odd, I wonder who rang you. Did he say his name?'

'No, he didn't.'

'I'll find out and sort it, one way or another. I thought I was getting on okay with H, but I must've pushed him a bit much.'

'I'll meet you for lunch.'

'Good idea. I'll have sorted it by then.'

Focused, his mind on the day ahead, he picked up his bag and was quickly out of the door and into the car. Pulling my dressing-gown around me, I poured another coffee from the pot and sat down in one of the old armchairs, welcomingly comfortable but not really pretty. I didn't know whether I liked the dressing-gown anymore. It'd been a bargain in a Laura Ashley sale. It had towelling on the inside and on the outside was a pink-flowered cotton fabric. Maybe it was too girly. I wasn't feeling girly.

Without mobile phones and instant texts, the only way of getting any early news was to be there at the Arts Centre where I could see Bob at our regular lunchtime haunt. I'd recently acquired a tiny old Fiat from my daughter, who needed a more reliable, not to say comfortable model. Not worth trading in, it was now providing me with some welcome flexibility. The winding, uneven island roads didn't encourage either speed or comfort, so I rattled along giving myself more time than necessary and trying not to think too much.

I usually liked driving around the island. The gentle slowness, the absence of traffic, and scenic beauty were a welcoming contrast to the frantic, traffic-filled commute through the unlovely industrial landscape of my not-too-distant experience, but today was different. My mind couldn't escape. That brutal, chilling image of H, slowly and deliberately informing Bob of his desire — his need — to kill his psychiatrist, wouldn't disappear. It didn't make sense. Nothing made sense. *Maybe it can't be made sense of… maybe we have to get real. Some things just can't be done. Why aren't the prison officers talking to Bob, warning him, taking it seriously? Maybe we should take this massive hint and just leave — leave the dungeon to be a dungeon, what's so special about us after all?* And so I prattled on and on to myself…

I was early. Sipping an indifferent cup of coffee, I placed myself with an eye on the door. Bob seemed bigger than my anxious remembering, as pushing through it and spotting me he gave a thumbs up.

'It's all fine, don't worry.'

'Yes, but is it okay? Was it real, the threat?'

'Yes, it was really okay, I asked the men if I should take it seriously, they said "Yes"… one or two said he'd have to get through them first.'

Laughing now, Bob said, 'Looking at them, that wouldn't have been difficult.'

'Okay, but really, what happened? What did you do, is it safe?'

'Well, you'll never guess, but the deputy governor has moved him to the Segregation Block, and they're finally managing it properly...'

As Bob told the story I began to relax. The prison was now protecting Bob, at least for the moment, but what if I hadn't had that phone call last night, what then? I wondered if it was the young officer who'd invited us to his wedding. I would've liked to thank him. Apparently, John was away and the morning meeting had been run by the deputy governor. Bob said he wanted H removed. He couldn't do his job, walk around the wing thinking he could be attacked at any moment. They all agreed the threat was real however. The probation officer, knowing much of H's gruesome history, was particularly insistent. The deputy governor had acted with impressive speed and management skill, and H was off the wing and encased in the Segregation Unit before Bob even reached the wing.

It was here, from his hard-won office, in the most tightly controlled area of all within this maximally controlled prison, that Bob operated an open-door policy, absurdly reflecting the best of modern management practice. So it was that three men came to ask that H be given another chance on the wing. It wasn't a delegation, they weren't lobbying. One by one they came into Bob's office—the man in the blue jumper, E, and an older man, long in the system. They understood H's situation, and they felt for him. If he didn't come back to C-Wing he faced a prison life of segregation and the notorious 'roundabout'—endless destabilising moves. 'I see myself in him', the older man had said, 'but he's got a chance here to straighten himself out.' The deputy governor too supported Bob. He told H the psychiatrist would visit the next day and report back to him, and he'd make the decision whether H could return. It was strong, decisive, wise action, leaving a way open for a solution.

The next day I was still worried as Bob got ready to leave for the prison, determined to see this man who'd planned to kill him. *Was he still planning? How could anyone be sure?* I recalled those sunken dead eyes, lifelessly skittering across his face. *How could Bob possibly be certain? This wasn't theoretical, Bob was testing his approach with his life, and I couldn't, wouldn't stop him by screaming* 'Tell the scumbag to get lost! I've had enough, it's not worth it!'

Instead I gave him a tight hug, saying pedantically, 'Take care.' I so wanted the day to be over, to be able to greet him with another pedantry of ours,

'How'd it go?' The physical threat was immediately all-consuming, but as the day progressed I allowed myself other thoughts. This was the pivotal moment, the absolute test. *If Bob's approach couldn't work with this man then would Bob have to admit failure and defeat? And then what next?*

But sitting on H's bed in the cell in the Segregation Unit, Bob found a man desperate to return. 'I can't do this anymore. I've got to get back. Got to sort my head out.'

Re-engagement

Later we chatted. It had been an exhausting day. 'Bob, how did you know it was safe?' Bob told me he was satisfied he could re-engage with H. The deputy governor had allowed him to return, so now H was back on the wing, and Bob's door, as ever, was open … would be open tomorrow. *Why, why, why would he want to kill Bob, the one person who was persistently, patiently trying to understand him and to help?* The glib, fearful, well-documented mantra 'addicted to violence' was never an answer. Later he was to confide … 'Strange thing to say but I am frightened of myself … I didn't want to see it … I couldn't have a conversation with anyone … all I knew was I had to attack them … that was my answer.'

'But you, you got a grip straightaway, you thought "there's something that made him the way he is …" you just kept digging "… after that little upset, I came back, and we started seeing each other again"' *'That little upset' was planning the murder of my dearest one.*

H had said to Bob: 'More came out that made me think more … now I've spoken with you about it … I've got no reason to be afraid of myself anymore … If I hadn't come here, I would have ended up with a record of killing three, four, five, anybody in the system who's got a bit of authority.' This was the absolute test of success or failure, and Bob was happy, revelling in the success.

The incident with H showed Bob's intention of turning the wing into a community where men wanted to help each other, as well as themselves, was beginning to work. I too could not help but feel more optimistic. Prison management, officers and men were all behind this peaceful solution, wanting both H and Bob to succeed. I wondered afresh whether the young officer who'd invited us to his wedding had been the anonymous caller who'd warned us.

Thinking of this crucial bit of compassionate management, when H was allowed back onto the wing, I remember a time when this same governor invited us to visit one of the new private prisons he'd been head-hunted to run. He gave us a personal tour. The prison was new, clean and shiny, with modern plumbing and the latest technological security. Designed to be a functional, efficient container, it was chilling. I could forgive the Parkhurst building, it reflected the age in which it was built. *This new building—was it hopelessly, brutally reflective of this age, the age into which I was born?*

A corridor led into a recreation area, and as the door was unlocked I saw a small boy. He looked about eleven, pale, lifeless, hopeless and afraid. There was a painful compassion in the Governors' face as he said, 'They shouldn't be here with the older prisoners, but there's nowhere else to send them. He's fifteen.' He'd done his best... there was a table-tennis table, but that was about all, and he tried to protect them, to keep them separate, but the prison was designed to run with fewer staff, and what the boys needed was attention, so much attention. *Was this how those C-Wing boys started off on their brutal careers?* I remembered E's earnest northern tones, *'If someone had taken an interest, none of this need have happened.'*

It was painful, our powerlessness.

CHAPTER 16

The Inspectorate Calls

HM Inspectorate of Prisons is a weighty body, and an inspection report a weighty matter. Mandated by Act of Parliament, it examines conditions within prisons and the treatment of prisoners, functioning independently of the Prison Service. Full reports are published on each prison every five years, shorter ones, half-way through. It was around this time we were expecting a full report following a recent visit to Parkhurst headed by His Honour Judge Stephen Tumim, the chief inspector, and a specialist healthcare inspector, a forensic psychiatrist who had visited C-Wing.

I was getting used to the calm after the storm over H, and was working in my office when Bob came in. He looked a bit upset.

'Whatever's the matter?'

'The hedge is all gone!'

'What do you mean, what hedge?'

'You remember, the one in the prison, with little pink flowers...'

I remembered it well, it was a welcome sight on that scary first visit, a 'trusty' prisoner had been tenderly clipping away at it. It was dense, and it must have been growing there for years.

'Whyever would they want to get rid of it?'

'There was a digger, they just ripped it up, it didn't take long... they were digging trenches, laying pipes, there's lots of building works going on...'

It was more than just a lovely hedge, it was the doomed 'canary in the mine', signalling a mess of thoughtless, unintended consequences in the wake of the long-planned roll-out of a previous administration's commitment to decent conditions for prisoners. An end to slopping-out and the start of time spent out of cells in purposeful activity required a mass of building works and new facilities. An ancient building like Parkhurst required more than most to implement all of the Woolf Inquiry's recommendations on the prevention of riots.

Even as all this finally got under way, I could see the new politics of crime rowing back from decency, and instead emphasising punishment, increasing sentences, reviewing tariffs. If I couldn't see then the effect this swirling eddy of new policies would have, I had seen the new in-cell loos: industrial-strength stainless steel, securely bolted to the concrete floor, they couldn't be smashed and used as weapons, for attack or self-harm. Lids and extractor fans, of course, were banished as security risks. I flinched at the thought of the smell. *I don't suppose Lord Justice Woolf ever thought decency meant living in a loo all day. Probably just that it would be nice to have a toilet in the room when prisoners returned to go to sleep, after all their purposeful activity during the day—but for all that, better than a bucket.*

The report

We were having a bit of a jolly in the supermarket with our daughter, who had come down for a precious stay, bringing her new baby. Planning a family feast, we had delightedly tossed treats in the trolley, and abundantly laden were on the way out when smashing into this lovely fun came John. Purposefully manoeuvring between the trolleys, he was grinning with a more-than-usual intensity. He knew our daughter, and at first I thought *That's nice he wants to welcome her,* but no. He told Bob: 'The inspector's report is out. They've got it in for you alright. You'd better have a look at it.' And he paused, almost hopping from foot-to-foot in anticipation. *Anticipation of what? What could possibly have caused this?* Stunned, I didn't want to notice it. Bob, silent, half-nodded at John, and started pushing the trolley away while I said something like, 'Bye John, got to get all this stuff home, mouths to feed and all that...'

'What was that all about?' was an equally stunned daughter's response, and driving home I tried to make some comforting sense out of it. 'John's just playing some schoolboy game, let's see what the report actually says... this inspector's a judge, a sensible fellow... rational, he has a liberal reputation. He did that hard-hitting report on prison suicide, after all... it's clear the men are changing, everyone knows what you do is working. The inspection team will have talked to the men.' Bob was not so sure. 'John was gloating. He thinks I'm toast.'

My wishful optimism evaporated. This was heavy… the reliably joyful prop of Bob's constant enthusiasm no longer there, I flinched at a freshly raw challenge: a reality I didn't want to see came crowding into my head. *It can't be that bad. We'll soon be home. A bit of a feast, and a good time… it'll be alright.* I see now how reality challenges weren't only for me and the men, but for the very Home Office itself, where mandated political ideas pushed constantly against pragmatic actualities. John too writhed in this sticky trap. *Surely he could, would somehow find a way to support Bob.*

It was early autumn and the next day on my walk I notice the gentle pink of nerines, which had waited patiently in bulbs all summer and were now bursting into gently waving life. I remember long-gone years, when my mother needed to protect hers from the harsher northern weather and delighted in giving me a precious bundle, along with a handful of fresh parsley from her ever-productive cold frame. *'It's full of iron', Susan,* she would say, and well, I don't know about iron but I was in need of a bit of steel, impervious to all these slings and arrows. *Had I managed to forge a pure enough steel that repulsed corrosion and deflected hurt? But then how steely did I want to be? Wasn't the point of all this to be able to remain human, and to hurt?* And so, I ruminated in painful circles as I closed in on a curious mix of acceptance and determination.

This time it was Bob who anticipated the clanging gate on my return, and was pouring hot water onto fresh grounds as I entered the kitchen. He was home early, shaken and serious.

'I've seen the report, it's peculiar. I'm the only person named and criticised. I can't understand it… I'd thought a professional… a psychiatrist, would be interested, would want to know… and John, he *knows* that C-Wing is calm, staff want to work there now… he knows it's safer… why aren't they pleased?'

'What does it say? What did this psychiatrist say to you when he visited?'

'Not a lot, I think he wasn't listening… I took no notice… the man seemed unreal, my job is to succeed with the men. As long as I have access it's fine.'

'Yes but what did he say?'

'I think he was just rude. A meeting was all arranged, but the day before it he pulled rank and called me out of a meeting with the psychologists. He said any idea the men are improving is "anecdotal, there has been no change". He was outraged, he was furious!'

'But hadn't he talked to the men?'

'He had, and they'd praised C-Wing and told him no alarm bells had been rung for the last two years. None at all! It's mentioned in the report. So why aren't they happy?' *Why indeed?* I breathed out an ocean of twanging hurt. There were so many nasty reasons for being what I felt to be gratuitously cruel.

Bafflement

Bob was baffled and so transparently real. I looked at him with such an ache. I couldn't protect him from this dismissive trampling over his work, his ideas, in which even common decencies appeared to be being ignored. He was still that young convincing idealist rushing to engage, to understand and to solve the most difficult of problems in human relations— *Why do we hurt each other?* My eyes could see him bathed in that summer light of oh so many years ago, the idealism of youth still clinging to him, energetically batting a fresh white ball. I reached for the cups and said, 'That coffee looks good, I think we need it.'

Bob was vulnerable, he had no power; no patronage to sprinkle, no promotions, research grants, powerful friends or esteemed publications were within his gift. If they felt like kicking him, they could. He didn't even have the minimal protection afforded by a formal contract. No, any power he had was so very different, the power to transform suffering through understanding; the opposite of coercive, it was a power that could only be offered, not imposed.

By now we'd managed to bring down our old sofa from up North. A relic from my parents' house, we'd had it re-covered in serviceable petrol blue Dralon®, and it had weathered many a mishap. However, it was still comfortable, and I liked its shape, elegantly long with narrow arms. Dralon was too functional for my taste, and I'd always had a dream that some time I might clothe it in tangerine pink velvet. Well, we were certainly in need of a bit of soft velvet at the moment.

'Here you are you lovely old thing and there's the milk, it's hot.'

'That's nice, thanks.' And so we relaxed, both drained and thoughtful in our comforting sitting-room on our old sofa, facing out to the garden and the sea beyond.

A few days later Bob, gnawing away at an attempt to understand, and quoting from a large psychiatric tome authored by the esteemed psychiatrist from the inspection team, declared, 'That's it, he thinks psychopaths are untreatable. If I'm right, he's wrong, and he's been barking up the wrong tree.' 'Bob, that really is too simple, too silly... what about professional support? Curiosity? Enquiry? There's an important issue here. He's top of the tree, he can't just be jealous!'

This wasn't just a bit of bad news. I felt instantly, sickeningly threatened. This was the ugly tip of a monstrous urge to stop Bob. *Fuelled by what? A mess of anger, ideology, politics, career advancement...* I couldn't tell. It was irrational, Bob was making the Prison Service safer. He was tackling men who'd been in solitary confinement for years, and he was cheap. Only part-time, he had already saved his fees in reduced drug costs. They knew all this, but of course they weren't looking. Bob's work had to be invisible, the men changing had to be invisible. *Perception is a funny thing... the impossible can't be happening. Serious psychopaths can't be transforming into ordinary humans. So, Bob must be pretending, and more than that they must demand, insist that he doesn't know what he is doing, absolutely doesn't know. And what of John? He knew about 'Salmon Code' procedures, he used them after all.* These were contractual obligations which enshrined notions of common decency and natural justice, allowing those about to be criticised to see, and respond prior to the publication of a report. Bob was an outside, self-employed specialist, and the code only applied to civil servants, but all the same it wasn't normal to name an individual who had no redress. No-one else was named, despite the documented increase in stabbings and serious assaults on other wings, the 'awful conditions for psychiatric patients in the hospital wing', and a suicide awareness group which had stopped meeting. *Singling out Bob's attempts to reduce violence for public ridicule looks like an attempt to slaughter a career.*

I only felt that despite being an ambitious and still-young Governor whose star was on the rise, John was having to collude in this personal attack. The *zeitgeist* was changing and Bob was an embarrassment whereas once he'd been a feather in John's cap. Contact with my sparky friend began to wither. It was becoming too difficult, the attempt at a jokey normality: we were digging in, retreating into an understanding I didn't want to share.

CHAPTER 17

A Breaking Storm

I began travelling to London quite a bit following up some of my old work, and Bob, well Bob was still eagerly amassing his evidence: the tapes, an audit of prescribing, of behaviours, of violence, of incidents leading to alarm bells. They were all heading in the right direction. True there was still the odd spat with some of the staff but generally it was workable. Bob too was travelling quite a bit, giving talks, enthusiastically explaining the basis of his work. Seasoned by now in many a crisis, I had learnt to ignore gathering clouds.

An escape

Then three prisoners from D-Wing escaped over the wall and were loose on the island. At first, I was slow to realise the arrival of an absolute storm: John after all had weathered such things before. Unconcerned, I remembered a previous escape. We'd been having an early supper with a cheery John and my sparky friend when his hotline rang. John knew the escapee of old and cursing him for all the trouble he was causing he'd sprung into decisive action, and the prisoner was found not long afterwards, having clung to the underside of one of the garbage trucks that removed the tons of Parkhurst rubbish. There had been reports, some sort of investigation, but John hadn't seemed troubled by it, indeed it had been the subject of hilarity.

So, I merely thought the three escapees would be quickly found, reports made, lessons learned, and normal life resumed. However, these were new times. Any facts available were being wound up into a dangerous hysteria, and the longer the men evaded recapture the more job-threatening criticism landed on the Home Secretary. Reporters swarmed the island and massed visitations of headquarters staff descended on the prison. A competing mix of accounts, intent on either lurid publicity, attacking comment or a defensive sifting of facts became an ever-more inflammable mix. As a toxic ball-tossing blame game began, a swirling colossus of reports, memos, investigations, interviews, articles, and news items began to drown all sense. The island itself seemed to be in lockdown. Helicopters flew overhead and what seemed the entire local police force created road blocks. Ferry ports were blockaded and mugshots of the escapees were everywhere. Warnings for residents to check garden sheds, outbuildings, barns, for signs of use and break-ins were constant. Rumours were rife, fuelling fearful panic. Island lanes and paths, normally full of cheerful ramblers, were deserted.

Bob seemed curiously unaffected. He was of course carrying on with his work. He'd noticed a bit more activity than usual at the gate. It took irritatingly longer to get through the airlock. I later read of the Director-General's irritation too. He'd sped down from London and was kept waiting outside in his car while earlier arrivals, the head of security and the regional director, were being processed. An unwelcome opportunity for the waiting reporters and the intrusive questions he couldn't answer.

On Bob's return that first evening, question after question tumbled out of me. 'What was it like in the prison? D'you know what happened? What are the officers like, have they said anything? What do you think, how dangerous are they? How's John?'

'Didn't notice much really, just got on with my work, I had a lot of appointments. Officers didn't say anything, and it's all a bit ridiculous really, they can't get off the Island. They aren't that dangerous, it's the C-Wing men who are. Didn't see John.'

'Well, I suppose the officers wouldn't discuss it with you anyway, they'd have to close ranks. There must have been some mistakes...' 'Yes, we'll see what happens.'

And see we did. Four days later the men were spotted by an off-duty prison officer trudging along a main road. Tired, cold and hungry, the two older men gave in. The youngest, in his early twenties, ran off over fields to the Medina estuary. Pursuers became rescuers as he floundered in the icy January waters, attempting an impossible swim.

Bit by bit news of how they'd managed such an extraordinary escape emerged. It was a surreal adventure story of skill, teamwork, planning, persistence, observation, courage... and luck. It was to have consequences far beyond what any of us could ever have anticipated. As I learnt of the incredible sequence these men had needed, I didn't think they ever believed they'd actually succeed. *Surely it had been an impossible dream for them, a project that gave them purpose, meaning and excitement, that used their brains and eased their boredom? It was a fantastical plan of great complexity, complete with an ending where they all flew away…*

I thought of my first frightening sight of that tall, so tall redbrick prison wall, with its bulbous overhang and razor-wire, designed to be incapable of climbing. They had somehow made a ladder kit by slicing up inch-thick metal rods, crafting suitable brackets and hiding the bits for later assembly. It would have needed to be excessively long and heavy to reach the top. They'd tied cable to the ladder to aid their descent to the ground outside. Cable is difficult to knot, especially in a hurry. They were lucky not to injure themselves as they hauled their bodies over and down to the earth far below. Lucky too that the CCTV seemed to have a blind spot, and it didn't flash up this unusual activity. *It must have needed the strength of all three to raise up the ladder, but how did they even get it to the wall?*

The huge and ugly inner perimeter fence made of thick metal mesh protecting a wide, barren no-man's-land wasn't alarmed. They couldn't have known they were in the only maximum-security prison that had yet to install geophones, but still it must have taken some strength and time to cut a large enough hole, and they were lucky that the CCTV seemed have patchy coverage, and the officers on duty in the Emergency Control Centre that evening were inexperienced, and that the lighting also suffered from insufficiencies. The hole in the fence was only discovered by a patrolling officer with a guard dog over an hour later. *How had they got to the fence?* With a master key, fashioned patiently, carefully, secretly, its shape informed by intense scrutiny of carelessly dangling keys. It was a classic old-fashioned escape aided by old-fashioned technology, old-fashioned buildings and a prison in a chaos of building works.

Reaction of the new Home Secretary

The escapers were to continue their prison careers. Not so those within the Prison Service, for this was not a daring prank, an extreme *Boys Own* adventure, to be laughed off once the men were safely re-incarcerated. No, it touched on the political fortunes of the newly appointed Home Secretary, Michael Howard, who it seems was bent on securing his reputation with a 'tough on crime, tough on criminals' strategy. A dramatic-headline grabbing failure of security in a flagship prison was finger-pointing dynamite, coming as it did only a few short months after the escape of five IRA prisoners from Whitemoor Prison in Cambridgeshire. Intense scrutiny fell on the Home Office,[1] the workings of the Prison Service and its executive. A creative reworking of accountability quickly emerged bolstered by all the might of political office and parliamentary privilege. This centred on the notion that operational matters concerning the running of prisons, including for preventing escapes (however ingenious or stemming from Government cutbacks they might be), rested with the Prison Service not it's highest accountable Minister-of-State. I later wondered did he ever reflect on his actions in sacking the Director-General, questioning the mere removal of John Marriot as Governor of Parkhurst, and doubling the escapers' tariffs or the despairing response of all concerned.

We watched in horror the unfolding of a horrible ending, as the might of political power became engaged in diverting culpability from the very person whose policies, actions and words were fracturing the careful accommodation between the incarcerated and those in charge of incarceration. John was caught in the crosshairs of an implacable political expediency. In Parliament, amidst a blizzard of comment and questions the Home Secretary rose and denounced him. With unusual intensity he declared, 'That man' was today being removed from Parkhurst and should never work in a prison again. The meaning of this was soundbite clear: an incompetent Governor had been sacked by a tough, efficient Home Secretary in the interests of public safety.

Years of endless memos and reports documenting the security risks involved in conducting major building works whilst keeping a top-security prison fully-functioning were all to be documented in the inevitable inquiry report: a colossus of detail, showing the impossible, chaotic managerial demands placed on the governance of Parkhurst. Staggered, I was to read of the 'blizzard of paperwork' which tied John to that huge desk for fifty hours every week. How had he remained cheerful, let alone connected, as he did, to the officers, the men, all the wing governors? I read too of his persistent stream of memos,

---

1. Prisons are now the responsibility of the Ministry of Justice not the Home Office.

reports and letters requesting funding for the more-than-obviously lacking security measures, geophones, dog patrols and CCTV improvements. All ignored in the engulfing bureaucracy of a seemingly overwhelmed headquarters.

These requests, and the accompanying bland responses, were carefully listed in an almost farcical eighty item appendix to the official enquiry report about the escape. No-one, I think, must have been more surprised by failure to act than the escapers, who were able to take an easy advantage. In the prison the officers were worried about John and talked to Bob. 'You're his friend, can't you speak to him? See if he's alright, go to the pub with him...?' We were worried too. How could this proudly cheerful man accommodate himself to such public exposure? Uncharacteristically, Bob was uncertain.

'I don't know Sue, they seem to think I can do something, that I can help... I'm not sure if he'd want me to...' 'They don't know what to say. They must be a bit frightened to actually ask you. Ring him up and meet him at the pub, he just needs to know that you know it's dreadfully wrong, and you care. Maybe it'll help a bit.'

Against all expectation and beyond all reasoning, Bob was still at Parkhurst and John had been removed, sidelined in a non-job in headquarters: a vicious blow that must surely have drained all his energy and optimism. No room now for those gleeful sparks of confident hilarity. It would be hard for Bob, for both of them.

'How did it go?'

'Not good. He didn't speak much, he's pretty depressed. He's having to commute to London. Parkhurst wasn't just a job, he loves the island life, community... his home. It was all a bit worrying. I couldn't do much...'

It was indeed a sad and dismal meeting between the two of them. Brutally insistent as this scapegoating of John was, it wasn't enough to quell the mounting questions as to the manner, and legitimacy of his removal. It became a continuing media discussion. An increasingly defensive Home Secretary arguing that operational matters were not his responsibility directed blame onto the Director-General himself. Refusing to resign, Derek Lewis was summarily sacked. The Home Office later found itself settling a claim for wrongful dismissal for a quarter of a million pounds. Beleaguered, John had no such redress. Howard's statement to Parliament about why John was being removed from Parkhurst was protected by parliamentary privilege and not admissible as evidence in any claim, a fact of which a legally trained Home Secretary must have been well-aware.

A miasma of gloom began to settle around the prison as edicts from above came crashing down. Bob, unwilling to think his precious work was under threat, kept going. The officers, he said, were being unusually helpful. C-Wing held prisoners were extremely difficult to place elsewhere. This just might be the saviour of Parkhurst's Category A status, and all the career opportunities that went with it. It now, of course, had all the long-denied security equipment needed, and logic reasoned everything could continue. So many people hoped so.

Reacting now to Bob's less cheery mood, I sensed the spiralling of gloom.

'How did it go today?'

'Oh well the piranha's had it.' Wound up and thinking he must be talking metaphorically, splintered thoughts hit. *Everything, it was all over… Maybe it's a relief, what do we do next?*

'Oh Bob, what do you mean, what's going on?'

'The piranha, don't you remember? On the wing in the sitting area.'

'Yes, the men fed it with guppies from the other wings, what about it?'

'The tank's smashed to bits… you remember R, the man with the square head?'

'Yes… I shook his hand at the tea party.'

'It was all a bit dramatic, he came down from the landings with a length of wood and just smashed it into the tank. It was actually quite dangerous, lots of glass splinters and a huge pressure of water.'

'Bloody hell, that's a bit significant isn't it? What's happening there?' And suddenly hungry I said, 'I think I'll have some toast and honey, do you want some?'

'Just some green tea, thanks.'

Smoothing chunks of butter far too thickly onto the toast, I said, 'Let's sit outside.'

A curious moment seemed to be upon us. Bob sipped his tea, I crunched my toast. I enjoyed the honey mingling with the butter. It added a soothing sweet softness to my crunching.

'Can you see that ship out there? Is it a tanker or the Brittany ferry?'

'I can't really tell, it's about the right time of day for the ferry, but it needs to get a bit nearer before we're sure.' *What was Bob thinking? What was I thinking?*

Did I want to see it… talk about it…? Feeling weary I stroked Bob's hand. *Was this going to be the beginning of the end?*

E… the man in the blue jumper… X… H… the men were being scattered, selected for disposal in the bowels of a regime's chilling lodgings. Wakefield, Whitemoor, Woodhill, Broadmoor, Rampton, Ashworth… a hierarchy of unpleasantness. The cages afforded an extreme isolation reserved for those at the top of the danger tree, there weren't so many of those; the control units, second order cages, where even socialising has to be earned; high-security hospitals, terminal lodgings for the incurably madly evil. Sadly, I hoped some of them might make Grendon — *There'll be a bit of a chance there. Even the ordinary high-security prisons might give them more of a chance, at least Bob's prepared them, they can talk about stuff…*

Bob had been thinking about R. 'It was a reaction of his to all the uncertainty. They're starting to move Cat A prisoners. It's not good. I'm giving a talk at the annual conference of the Royal College of Psychiatrists soon, maybe they can help. They surely can't close the only unit doing this work.' An inch, a sliver of hope wormed its way into my brain. I faintly realised how wearily depressed I had become. John's removal had sliced through my necessary optimism. *Was it only a pretence I'd been nurturing all these years of the power of humanity, kindness and trust? But just maybe we could do* something… *they must have some influence, and they must surely be the ones to see the value of Bob's work?*

Now I have an even sadder clear-eyed despair as I look back on a remorseless draining of kindness, compassion and truth from decision-making. Was it twelve times the man charged with overseeing our system of imprisonment refused, on national TV, to say whether or not he had threatened to overrule Derek Lewis concerning Lewis' decision to remove John to other work rather than suspend him? We'd gazed at the screen as the awesomely fixed, carefully worded response, 'I didn't instruct him' attempted to deflect *Newsnight*'s Jeremy Paxman as he repeatedly but unsuccessfully sought a direct answer from Howard as to whether he had threatened to overrule Lewis. I had laughed, clutching at the comedic, insistent absurdity in relief, my amusement soothing and softening the sad implications of the words I so didn't want to notice.

Truth from nonsense

'Oh Bob, it's too ridiculous.'

But Bob, for once less cheery than me, wasn't seduced by the comedy of it. 'It's not funny. John's destroyed. The facts seem to be... what can I say?... It's so damaging...' There was an agony of distress in Bob's sad rational words, his long arms hard clasped around one knee as he bent intently forward, seemingly protecting what he could of himself. A weary blight took lightening hold and my own arms felt weak, helpless as the knowing sadness struck. And so I turned to concentrating on the hope that Bob's fellow professionals had influence and could provide useful endorsement.

This time his audience was a conference of psychiatrist colleagues, and he was travelling there with the intrigued support of an eminent professor and a well-known consultant. Tackling violence and treating personality disorders were becoming the new cutting edge in psychiatry. Big debates on treatability—whether it was a lifelong disorder, whether people were born with the condition—were just revving up. No-one was even attempting what Bob was doing. No-one was able to show actual films of unique therapy with clearly dangerous people.

Rekindling my optimism I said, 'It's encouraging they've asked you to speak. Surely it means something... they know about C-Wing... Bloody hell, talk about unique, what you can show them! They *must* grab at it... set up proper research and training... teaching...'

Bob was once more off to deliver his message, to show his work, to expose his therapy and thinking for all to see and discuss, but this time it was not to an assembly of cynical prison governors or weary civil servants, defending themselves from the pain of compassion. I remembered the now cruelly crushed optimism of that first conference, where an ebullient John and enthusiastic Bob had pushed themselves into the consciousness of a Prison Service. Driving Bob to the ferry I was all encouraging chatter, and Bob too was confident. 'Don't worry... it'll knock their socks off.'

Definitely a suit job this: I had suggested the light grey we'd bought for a wedding, not the dark Parkhurst one. *He'll have a good time,* I thought happily. The unfolding of a much larger picture, the fracturing of trust, the emboldening of the powerful to ignore the powerless I put from my mind. And he did have a good time. A beaming thumbs-up greeted me as he reached the end of the walkway from the ferry on his return. It had knocked their socks off! The president of the Royal College of Psychiatrists no less had bounded down the central gangway saying 'We have influence, we can help! Write to me, we can stop C-Wing closing.'

So Bob did, with information, with statistics, with documents. The responding absolute silence said more than any letter. Bob was cast off on his own. Our little bubble of hope was quickly, and ferociously, burst.

CHAPTER 18

Resignation

When it came it was not a decision, it was an angry howl. Bob, home from London and a meeting of the SUSC, crashed into the kitchen… 'One man is banging a pencil into his head, another is burning his foot in a fire he made in a wastepaper basket… they need to be on the unit, but they won't let them come. They're taking my patients away, they're saying all Cat As have to go as Parkhurst is now Cat B, but then they move them to a Cat B prison with a special Cat A unit, which is what we have here! There's not many left. The SUSC is under orders. It's political. I have to protest somehow… it's wrong, it's stupid, it's unnecessary… it was working! I've resigned in protest. I had to!'

''Course you bloody well did!' My outrage matched Bob's fury. Determinedly and still furious Bob penned an open letter to the Home Secretary and sent it to the *Guardian*.

'The harshness of your prison policy has ground my therapeutic endeavours to a sickening halt', he began, a lyrical starkness that made me weep. Whether this hit a nerve we were never really to know. The *Guardian*'s response to the letter was instant. The telephone rang. 'Yes, I'll get him', I said, remembering that meeting in the *Guardian* offices to discuss Bob's column 'In the Prison Psychiatrist's Chair.' I had sensed their fear for him, for whilst sharing Bob's values they knew rather more than us the crushing realities of power, and as we turned to leave the editor had caught my eye, saying, 'Keep an eye on him, won't you?'

I made a coffee while I listened, trying to get a sense of what they wanted. I could hear only Bob's animated passion about the folly of it all. Dunking a bit of old, hard toast smothered in butter into my coffee, I was nervously moody… *Oh this is all too much I'm getting fat as well.*

Bob put the phone down. It had been a long chat. 'They're going to run with it in tomorrow's *Guardian* and want an embargo on it.'

'What? What does that mean?'

'Well, I think it means they'll print it tomorrow, and probably run an article on it, so they don't want me to circulate it 'til then. It's good, it will get some publicity. They're sending a photographer. I'll meet him in Newport.'

'I'll tell the kids to buy it tomorrow, they'll want to know. I hope they print it all. And well, at least we'll have more time to see them...'

We'd had a bit of a night. It had been too sudden: I wanted to be there, supporting his lonely exit. I couldn't help thinking about that last journey of his, leaving Parkhurst a final time. When he came back, I kept poking him with questions, as if knowing more would somehow soothe my anguish.

'What did they say, what did anyone say?'

'Well the men, they shook my hand.' There were only about five of them left now 'They knew of course it was coming way before I let myself know. One said I'm surprised you lasted so long. It was curious really. They were steadying themselves for re-immersion into a brutal world. I'd already gone in their minds...'

'And the officers?'

'Nothing, really... there weren't many about.'

'Didn't anyone help you? It's a long way...'

That first trek slid into my mind. *The locking and the unlocking, the ugly wire mesh, the concrete paths—even bleaker now with an absent hedge—the sliding airlock at the gates, but then a bouncy John was smoothing the way, and an eager Bob was happily anticipating his work ahead, the most difficult challenge in psychiatry laid out for him to solve.*

'No, it was a bit tricky, I had to pull my chair with the boxes on it. One of the wheels came off, no way I was going back for it...'

'Didn't anyone say anything?'

'Well when I was in the final airlock at the gate the young officer controlling it shouted down, "Someone pissed you off then?" Yes, I said, Michael Howard!'

'Oh Bob...'

'Sweetheart, I wanted to help and they wouldn't let me...'

I had no words, only tears and some gulping hugs. We put the chair in the garage, waiting transfer to the tip. And the left behind wheel? I supposed it met with a similar end. The left-behind thoughts in men's minds I hoped could not be so easily junked.

Headline day

Bob was up early, eager to see if the full text of his letter had been printed. He'd laid out in careful detail his absolute objections to current policy, and its inherent futility. He wanted them all to know.

Well, know they did... It was the front-page, headline article: 'Jail shock for Howard... leading prison psychiatrist resigns...' Bob's letter, citing the harshness of Government penal policy, was there alongside his photograph. He hadn't removed his crumpled grey anorak. It matched his thick mass of unruly hair. There was a sad determination in his gaze. His compassionate eyes were sombre, infused with the cruel clarity of what he knew. He looked compelling. He *was* compelling.

Bob still had his porridge, of course, followed by thick slices of toasted bread while he read the pages spread out on the table before us. This wasn't anything he had anticipated. He was surprised, elated and very cheerful. 'Look Sue, they've put it all in, and more, it's great... I wonder what will come out of it?'

I wondered too. Unlike Bob, I was anxious; quite a private person, I flinched from exposure. Many people might well hate what Bob was saying. Home Office policies, after all, were designed for popular appeal. I wasn't feeling brave, and sought to summon up anger to douse my fear. *This was an opportunity to speak truth to power, it had to be used... it really was right.* So I chuntered on to myself, whilst nervily anticipating something nasty.

It wasn't long before we experienced the power of a mass media headline. The phone kept ringing. The answering machine was full of requests. Letters forwarded from an efficient *Guardian* dropped noisily through our brass letterbox. Flowers arrived. I morphed into a secretary. Surprisingly there were no nasties. Instead, there were invitations to talk, a raft of supporting letters in the *Guardian* and direct personal letters of thanks and encouragement. It was overwhelming, this flood of kindness, this understanding. An unfamiliar and unnerving mixture of sorrow and delight hit me as I allowed myself to realise the extent of our isolation: it had been a lonely battle, but I was, we were both intact, and now was I feeling something like relief?

What had I said those few years ago? 'If it will work there it will work anywhere.' Well it had *worked there, but now it wasn't going to be allowed to work anywhere.*

John gone, and now Bob gone. How could this be allowed to drain such lifeblood from an organization created in the service of the public good? All this kindness, however—all this need—was disturbingly challenging. Our lime-green kettle did much good service in the production of strong coffee as Bob and I sat on our old sofa reading letters, such piles of letters: from families, sufferers, prisoners, colleagues and friends. *Could a fresh new template be emerging out of the flurry generated by this headline?* It began to rekindle our battered determination. *We mustn't allow this valuable footprint to be drowned in mud, sealed over, and rendered invisible.*

CHAPTER 19

Panorama

The aftermath of John's removal and Bob's resignation continued to be on the radar of newshounds wanting quotes and comments on stories of the day: their reputations seemed to have staying power, the one for his humanity, and the unfairness of a public pillorying, the other as the recklessly-outspoken liberal psychiatrist, so it was not altogether surprising when Bob said one day, 'John wants me to go over, he's got a reporter from *Panorama* there.'

Panorama, the BBC's flagship documentary programme, with a reputation for fearless, accurate reporting. I was impressed. *Should be interesting… wonder who the reporter is?* 'Interesting' was to be the least of the epithets I later used to describe what followed John's last ever assistance to him: later that day it was an excitedly cheery Bob who burst into the kitchen, throwing his coat down on the nearest available chair—'Well that was something! Could be good, this!'

I'd had a desultory afternoon of sorting my desk and clearing up a bit. Housework always became an irritant, both useless and necessary, and anyway, I wanted excitement too: suddenly cross, I muttered rather too loudly, 'What was? What's going on now? Bob, can't you be clear for once—what did they want?'

Tom

Bob looked at me, a bit surprised. He was bringing good news after all. 'What's the matter? Come and sit down and I'll tell you all about it.' 'Oh alright, who did you meet then?' We sat at the table in the kitchen. I'd just cleared it and it was slightly damp from the dishcloth, but I couldn't pretend I wasn't interested, and my crossness vanished as I heard that Bob had met Tom Mangold. I rated him. He was *the* face of *Panorama*, a well-known, hard-hitting master of well-researched reporting. He let the facts speak. 'So why was he there, what's he investigating? What's the programme he wants to make?'

'Not sure really, prisons, prison reform... that sort of thing, but he was very interested when I told him about the tapes. He's coming back next week with his producer, they're going to look at the tapes. Maybe this is the way to get the work looked at and properly evaluated', Bob carried on, 'that's what the men wanted, to let people know, to educate, to change things. They were brave you know, facing it all. Maybe this will make it alright, to have been worth it...' I suddenly felt an exceptional tenderness for this man who was still hurting, both from the cruel fracturing of the trust he had with the men, and the responsibilities he'd been prevented from pursuing. *Whoever else in this peculiar world would feel pain, rather than relief, on being prevented from talking to serial killers?*

Sadly, grim faces of the men in C-Wing crept into my view. *Where were they now? How were they now?* My thoughts, my feelings were all getting too uncomfortable. In an attempt at normality, I stood and smoothed Bob's lovely curly messy hair saying, 'Let's wait and see what they think. We'll have to be careful.'

I was thinking about the *Guardian* reporter's visit just two or three years before. We'd had bean soup while we more-than chatted, it was an intensive seminar: opinion-writing investigative journalists have a wide overview, and a questioning detachment, that was challenging, being rooted in the reality of a diversity of human encounters. *There was a great deal more than intellectual theories in their probing approach, and there were similarities with Bob's clinical approach: the human interest, the questioning, the linking to an over-arching model, but the underpinning purpose, of course, so very different. Theirs was to the primacy of their audience's interest, Bob's to the primacy of his patients' treatment.*

Anxiously wondering how best to protect Bob, to protect myself, I said, 'It wasn't good after those articles in the *Guardian*...' 'No, but it all blew over, and they did listen, it was pretty accurate. It got it out there. Lots of people read them. Remember all the letters?' 'Well, let's wait and see what they're like this time...'

Some of those past heart-clutching brain-splintering moments hit me again. I didn't want any more. I wasn't feeling brave, but I knew both that the tapes mustn't be allowed to wither away, unseen, unheard and unexamined, and that I'd dredge up some energy from somewhere. Bob was of course certain. It was the compact he'd made. The purpose of filming was so the tapes were used to throw as large a light as possible on the causes of, and the solutions to, extremes of emotional distress, abuse and torture. He busied himself sorting and documenting his archive. I fluttered around, 'It's all confidential, you can only show the ones that have written permissions.' 'Of course, don't worry, I've got them safe.'

The next week they arrived. Instantly recognisable, Tom was taller than I'd anticipated, my image to date being only of his head and shoulders filling a television screen. Whilst being friendly and interested, he exuded an extreme air of confident authority. *Working for a BBC flagship documentary programme must magically open doors all over the world,* I reflected. Bob's greeting was animated and our room, the largest one where Bob had his piano, soon filled with chat as two confident men batted around their differing agendas, then we settled to look at the tapes. Unlike Bob I was on twitchy alert.

It is, of course, riveting. I notice professional antennae quivering, as the producer looks at the reporter, and the reporter looks at the producer. The film is technically poor, a fixed single-angle shot, and amateur technology, but all an irrelevance against the overwhelming authenticity of the sight, the words: E is first up, his big frame and northern accent oozing a dreadful reality. Bob is giving a running commentary...

'That's it, did you hear that? It's astonishing... that's the evidence they are changing!'

They understood what Bob was saying, maybe even agreed, but I could see that wasn't the point, and was worried. For them it was astonishing, unique television, the rarest of scoops. It showed a dungeon hell and in it the close-up faces of killers, always the object of dread fascination. There was also Bob, who could talk and looked good.

So began the first of these defining conversations: the producer, a calm, professional man, explained how he could use the tapes alongside Bob and his explanations; Bob was enthusiastic, and, as the discussion progressed, I noticed from my careful perch at the back of the room their growing understanding of the importance of what Bob was trying to do, and perhaps, despite a professional distancing, some admiration. I understood distancing — after all, I was doing it myself, trying to remain detached from the lure of public acclamation, to keep our eye on the 'real ball', as Bob and I were to painfully discuss, but for them what wasn't there to be enticed by? Bob was a kind, charismatic, authoritative and captivating speaker, with a rare vocational passion, and it wasn't just words with him, either, he was a doer, and the tapes were showing this. Derek

Lewis, the former Director-General of the Prison Service, when authorising research and evaluation, had put in a supporting memo, 'Anyone who meets Dr Johnson can't help being impressed by his infectious enthusiasm.' *Maybe, just maybe, this was an opportunity to get done what the controversially sacked director had failed to manage, a way to avoid the fierce temper of an ever-more austerely managed prison regime, and allow plain truth to filter into the public domain.*

Wanting to be hopeful, I began to trust their integrity. They were, after all, part of a quality organization, producing programming in the public interest. So many chasing thoughts merged with pounding feelings as I sat back, almost unnoticed on the edge of the purposefully animated group.

'Be a great help if we took the tapes today, we can get on with it.' My reaction was instant. 'Absolutely not. They are confidential. There has to be a contract, and safeguards.' My words crashed into the agreeable, agreeing conversation. Bob was quick too. 'Sue's right, we can't move without a legal agreement.' We were serious, and what we were offering was alarmingly serious. They both knew it, and began to reassure us. 'Of course, I'll set up a meeting with the legal buffs and the *Panorama* director.' My twitchiness began to subside. I was reassured by the quick response and confident authority. It was only later I realised how influential this reporter, presenter and writer actually was.

Our demands and requirements

And so it started. We took non-negotiable demands to that first meeting. The *Panorama* offices were extensively open plan, bustling with self-aware important activity. I was surprised at the number of people telephoning, writing, chatting. It was clearly a huge enterprise; the head of all this was another hugely confident man. Their absolute rule was the sanctity of editorial control. Nothing could impinge on that, so our demand to have prior view of all the clips they would be using, as well as a veto in the patients' interest on the final film, took some arguing. This was later to prove crucial, not only for Bob, but for the BBC. Contracts negotiated, a schedule of filming was agreed. *So what to wear?* Surprisingly his navy Parkhurst suit was still holding out despite its hours on that ugly office chair. *Padded seat and arms had helped,* I supposed, *and there was little sign of shiny wear, but there remained the question of his tie. In Parkhurst long ties were a potential strangling invitation, and Bob had always worn a bow tie. Prison officers had pre-knotted black ones secured under the collar by thin elastic.*

A bow tie wouldn't do, it was a too iconically 'shrink'-shrieking message, I told Bob. 'Okay, whatever you think, I can practice my double Windsor knot. I don't want a boring one though.' 'No, of course not, just elegantly understated...' It wasn't easy, this tie selection business. I realised I had no clue about the sartorial messaging of ties. *Shiny, wide, thin, dark, light, patterned, striped, plain... whatever did these useless strips of cloth mean?* Bob of course just wanted the brightest, most cheerful. We enlisted the understanding help of our fashionable son-in-law. 'No problem, we'll go and look in Armani.'

It was a happy distraction from my looming worries, that little shopping trip. Armani is understatement to perfection. I noticed the carefully discreet assistant's amusement as the group of us argued over a tie. 'They're all a bit dull', pronounced Bob. 'This one's interesting, it's different.' The tie selected was made from a soft chenille fabric, and slightly darker than petrol blue, had a scattering of tiny white stars. Bob liked the fabric, and conceded to our delight at finding the perfect one. This tie was to have a number of outings as we plunged into the production whirlwind of a television documentary being made. Lights, cameras, sound equipment, crew, producer and presenter poured into our home for the first interview with Bob. I was relieved when a black cloth was set up behind him, so they weren't filming bits of our home, bits of our life. Bob later revealed he too felt protective of our privacy, and had discussed the background with the producer. It actually made for more powerfully-focused television.

BBC studios

That was a gentle location compared to the specialist, multiple-split-screen facility London studios we were now heading for. We were about to see the first clips of the men, his patients, and Bob's reaction was to be filmed. On the train journey to London, I fretted anxiously, wondering what they'd extracted from the tapes. *Would it all hold up, weren't we just riding a tiger?* Looking at the sky through the train window an image of a hovering hawk, its vibrating wing-feathers spread against the sky, flashed into my head. I'd seen it the day before. It was using the invisible air to support its determined purpose. *What was our invisible air, what was supporting our purpose?*

'Can we still pull the plug if it's not right?'

'Don't worry, let's see.'

See, we certainly did. The studio was huge, dark, technical. Bob sat on a stage, his familiar profile small against the cinema sized screen beside him. He looked smart, professional, authoritative. Sitting facing him, the presenter ran through some questions. Bob nodded, calmly prepared. Suddenly the vast screen filled with faces, each one allocated its own space in a monstrous grid, almost aping prison windows. The image was shockingly powerful. I recognised each face, but together, face after grim face, the cumulative effect was mesmeric and frightening. They looked unmistakably dangerous. I was shocked by the power of the images, and hoped this wasn't to be the over-arching message. I'd met those faces, but not like this. I'd seen individuals, terrifying, yes, but also desolate, hurting, struggling to be more than, and better than they were. The media people could slice things any way they chose, we'd have to be careful somehow. I wasn't feeling comfortable.

Then Bob started to speak, his kind understanding eyes a compelling, reassuring contrast. The faces became individuals, as one-by-one, extracts of his extraordinary conversations with them emerged onto the screen. He talked: explaining, describing, dissecting these courageous encounters, where fearlessly he was drilling down into the heart of the violence in the hearts of these men. It was the knowledge Bob wanted out there. Relieved, I was also apprehensive. The challenge to public perceptions was colossal. He was showing that violent offenders were also traumatised victims.

On the train home the carriage was empty, so we were able to chat through my rumbling fears, but in the end it was always starkly simple: we had to let this truth be seen. I remembered what E, the big man said: *The truth's gotta come out, don't it.*

We chose to trust the integrity of the production team, and I couldn't back away out of discomfort, so we continued with the project, Bob certain it needed to be out there whatever the backlash. Bracing myself, I began anticipating arguments to come, not knowing how futile a protection my scrawled thoughts would be. It began to feel exciting. Bob did location shots. The production team scoured the landscape to find a hilly vantage point from where, looking down, outlined by its crookedly looping walls, the prison could just be seen. I was surprised by its extent. Close up, of course, I'd seen only the immediate immensity of the walls, and the tortuous path to the innards of C-Wing.

The hill was the closest to Parkhurst the production team would ever get. Repeated requests for interviews, or just responses to questions, were ignored, even offensively so. On one occasion, after waiting and waiting, agreed arrangements were rudely denied. I imagined the utter offence to dignity, status, and authority, and the waste of an expensive production team's precious time. *Why was there such animosity towards a well-respected presenter from the BBC asking reasonable questions in the public interest?* The team was undoubtedly shocked. This prestigious public organization always got a hearing. It didn't make sense. I, on the other hand, was so used to such casual, controlling nastiness from the Prison Service that I wasn't at all surprised, and only really noted the extent of their outrage, but it proved to be a clear pointer to what was to come.

A date is set for the broadcast

The date for the broadcast was set for Monday the third of March, the day before my birthday. 'We'll stay in in London', pronounced Bob happily. 'It'll be a bit of a jolly... I promised Tom a bottle of Krug.'

Spectacular publicity was in preparation as the might of *Panorama* swung into action. There was to be a two-page article the day before in the Sunday papers, advance review copies and interviews set up. I heard Tom himself say he thought this might well be the most important documentary he'd ever made. All was set for a huge impact.

CHAPTER 20

The High Court

It was Friday, almost the start of the weekend and the London jolly, when around half-four in the afternoon the phone rang. Significantly, it was not quite the end of the working day. I was pottering about in the kitchen. Through the open door I heard Bob's shock as he answered. 'What?! On what possible grounds?' I clutched at an instantly thudding chest and knew I was still on total nervy high alert. 'What now?! What the bloody hell now?!'

An injunction

And it was a pretty, bloody 'now': the Home Office had been granted a hearing to obtain an emergency injunction. They wanted to stop the *Panorama* programme being aired. We had to be in the High Court in The Strand in Westminster on Monday morning. Accusing Bob of breaching the Official Secrets Act, patient confidentiality, and failing to inform the Prison Service, they were also threatening prosecution. They wanted the tapes destroyed. We had two days to prepare — to find documents, to seek legal advice, to obtain professional advice. This aggressive thunderbolt had been deliberately left to the last possible minute. We stared at each other.

'Bloody hell, Bob.'

'Yes it is.'

'We'd better have some coffee.'

'The BBC want us to be at the offices first thing tomorrow, bringing all the documents we have that could be useful. Memos, that sort of thing. They're booking a train, a hotel, and sending a car.'

My fury began to outpace my nerves, any weariness vanquished. 'It's rubbish, it's bullying. I'll look through the boxes. There are the memos to John, you absolutely told them. They'll be there, we didn't chuck anything, we never do.' I was right, I did and could find what we needed. Plodding through the boxes and through the night I was astounded by Bob's foresight. He'd even followed up the memos, insisting they be sent on to head office.

The next day, entering those *Panorama* offices once more, it seemed less buoyant, chillier. The chattering busyness was absent — it was a weekend after all — and I had the distinct feeling we were being minded, almost captured. The BBC's lawyers were searching for a way through... contract law, employment law, intellectual property rights, copyright, duty of confidentiality, Official Secrets, public interest... the solicitor was interrogating Bob with question after question. I couldn't tell how relevant they all were, all I saw was the lawyer writing and writing, writing it all down.

A huge weariness overcame me as I watched Bob in the claws of what suddenly seemed a terrible vengeance. Had his very public resignation hit a nerve that led to this? My brain was in an overdrive of anxious thoughts. How could we battle such persistent, cruel irrationality? We were, after all, relying on the BBC and its lawyers. *Maybe we have to pull out... Was it time to get our own advice?* Bob and I needed to talk, and we needed to sleep. We were both exhausted. It wasn't the time to say the wrong thing...

My sense of capture continued. We were driven to the hotel and shown our room. 'You can eat in the hotel. Best not to talk to anyone. A car will pick you up in the morning. Have a good night.' The door closed behind us, momentarily shutting out the oppression, the demands. My relief at being able to hug Bob was immense. That boring hotel room was briefly a haven, and I suddenly thought of my twin brother's daughter, a high-flying lawyer in a top-ranking city firm. She was feisty, clever and socially aware, and I absolutely trusted her and her ability. Bob strode to the telephone. 'Let's hope she's at home and has time.'

Time was of course the big one. We only had Sunday to sort it. She came straight over. We talked and talked, discussing the dangers to Bob, his reputation, his professional status if he were to pull out or if he were to fight and lose. It was perilous either way. Listening to her lawyerly brain dissecting the issues, it became clear we were enmeshed in a battle between two mighty institutions. The BBC's justification for all those licence fees was its ability to deliver accurate, fearless, impartial broadcasting in the public interest. Its independence from external pressure an absolute necessity. The Home Secretary's necessity was ensuring the safety of prison regimes. Nothing could or should be allowed to stand in the way of this. But right now it seemed that the public good was becoming synonymous with the will of the Home Office, using the Official Secrets Act as justification.

An affidavit

'They'll be constructing your affidavit from the documents, and all you've said, to present to the judge. The legal bits, the memos, the permissions, are all on your side, but he needs to accept your professional view. The affidavit will be protecting the BBC's interests, which might be yours but might not. I'll need to see it.'

We didn't have a very comfortable night. The beds in that type of mid-range hotel were always too small, and replacing the sea was a background hum of traffic, air conditioning, grumbling pipework and the odd screeching siren. Still, we felt relief, we'd got back some control. We'd take a view in the morning.

The car arrived at a reasonable time, and we were waiting, bags packed. It felt like an escape. Walking into the office once more, it was Sunday-morning deserted, except for a group of men in suits, urgently, importantly chatting. They waved Bob into a glass sided office where I recognised the lawyer from yesterday. I was of course invisible. The chatting group was animated, and I thought I heard mention of top level discussions between the Home Office and BBC.

Then the large, important man glanced round and noticed me. My presence became frighteningly visible, and suddenly out of his bubble of control he rapidly declared, with a determined emphasis, 'I didn't say that. That didn't happen. Understood?' A bit baffled, I didn't take much notice, thinking, *Well of course... levers of power and all that.* It was only later I realised its possible significance, and why any mention had to be so utterly denied, but for the moment I was only concerned with the looming High Court hearing next morning, and how to protect Bob. Saying hello to the group, I pushed past and into the office to where Bob was sitting, leafing through papers. 'This is the affidavit', he said, 'it will take a bit of reading.' It was a lengthy, complex, detailed document. The BBC's lawyer had worked hard, but it didn't sound like Bob, and some of the sequencing and the reasoning were wrong. It seemed to me more like an after-the-event, lawyerly justification. Injunctions, I now understand, are usually granted as staying orders so a proper court hearing can be arranged, and this affidavit was preparation for that.

All these wider implications escaped us as we concentrated on the immediate threat, the court hearing next morning: Bob's testimony had to reflect the truth, his integrity... with an uncharacteristic attention to detail, he was absolutely focused. 'I'm stating here that the programme won't cause prison riots. I have to see the actual programme that's going out. I can't be cross-examined on that if I haven't seen it.'

There was immediate resistance. 'You've seen everything we're using of the prisoners. That backs it up...' It was an issue of control, and maybe they were nervous of his reaction—would he pull the plug? These important decision-makers were meeting some of that inner steel that enabled Bob to do the work they were attempting to air. The tussle didn't last long. Instructions were given, and after a welcome coffee we trooped off for the viewing.

It was a powerfully immersive and emotive opening. There was my Bob, surrounded by stacks and stacks of tapes and the men's faces. The programme had its quota of required impartial balance and the team had interviewed other psychiatrists and psychopaths and gave a voice to the victims. Bob was satisfied. 'It's the men's faces that are so crucial. You can see what they were... how they were changing, and then the change. It's so important to see it.' It was true the faces were real, and their struggles pulled me in. It wasn't just horror, it was transformation too. I hoped an audience could see this, and the men. *Was their courage in facing themselves still intact?*

As I watched the figure of a psychopath under alternative treatment appeared. His face was fuzzed out, his very person denied. *Was his face too dangerous, infectious even? Or did he not deserve to be seen, was that it? Or were the public too vulnerable to be exposed?* I wondered if he'd even been asked. *Maybe everyone was too frightened of a vengeful public to show the truth.* His words were a doleful, familiar and unreassuring mantra. 'I will always be a psychopath, but have learned tools to control my triggers.' Exhausted with the watching, the tension and the thinking, I squeezed Bob's hand. We still had tomorrow to get through, but then what? I wanted some gentle calm, some normalcy, some fish and chips even. I didn't want to play with these big boys any more.

Back in the office I picked up our bag, and Bob said, 'We're staying at Sue's niece's tonight, can the car take us there? It's not much further than the hotel.'

It was an unpleasant surprise. They didn't like it, and tried to persuade us to stay in the hotel. *Needing to keep an eye on us, they're on edge too; unfamiliar with not having control, and having to trust,* I thought. I was angry. *We aren't their prisoners, we just need to get away.*

'The car will pick you up at six in the morning.'

It was a relief to step into the welcoming home of family. My niece had just fed her new young baby, and I followed her husband upstairs where he was gently settling the softly snoozing baby into his little cot. I bent and stroked the tiny head. His would be a cherished life. The unwelcome faces of the men assailed my brain as I returned to the kitchen... *What ugly cruelty had welcomed them into the world? Just maybe, this programme will be the start of a solution...*

And so we started, sitting round the table eating a takeaway and a lemon tart, with what were to be the first of many cups of coffee. Her lawyer brain was on full alert, and I was staggered how quickly she leafed through the affidavit, scribbling down numbered points. It was a trained, incisive, professional mind. And then came the questions, and after that the pronouncement: 'We have to start again. Write a new one, that Bob can sign. This is a BBC defence, it doesn't defend Bob or his professional practice, sufficiently.'

What had I said a few years ago? 'You'll need your wits about you in the morning', but this time, this morning, he faced an even bigger attempted assassination of his career, his reputation and finally of his very liberty. Bob, his doctor training still working, and his exhaustion absolute, was soon fast asleep. Upstairs, the study was lined with thick legal files, and heavy reference texts. Switching on the computer, she brought in another chair and placed fresh A4 notepads and sharpened pencils on the desk in front of us. By now it was dark, and the curtains were drawn. We had so much work to do, and so we started...

'I first entered Parkhurst in July 1991 at the invitation of John Marriott to work as a consultant psychiatrist in C-Wing...' Questioning, laughing, chatting, writing, we worked through the night, pausing to feed the baby, make coffee, and eat toast. It was a roller-coaster of prompted knowledge, sifted and accurately documented. I knew what Bob had said, what safeguards he'd insisted on, what he'd written, what he thought, what memos existed, what permissions. I constructed a chart documenting all the public talks and the many times E's video was seen. Finally, by five-thirty in the morning, we were satisfied we had an accurate, compelling narrative that Bob could testify was true. Light was dawning, and the birds were chattering as I woke him up. 'We've done it, this is what you can sign, not the other.' Quickly dressing, he read it over coffee and toast. Nodding 'Yes', he was looking relieved. 'I'll finish it off in the car.' I handed him the tie, ludicrously thinking it might work some magic on this outing.

The driver was early, and there was a rapid knocking on the door. I hoped it wouldn't wake the baby. *Good job I don't wear make-up,* I thought grumpily, *they haven't given me time.* Too tired to be nervous, I slumped tightly against Bob in the roomy car as he read the new affidavit.

We were offered coffee as we entered the still-quiet offices once more. Bob, holding the affidavit, handed it over to the lawyer saying, 'This is the affidavit I will sign. I can support every word.' A stunned, worried silence greeted this pronouncement. It was, of course, an ultimatum: there wasn't time to discuss or alter it. The barrister had to have it straightaway. As the lawyer quickly read it through, I detected signs of relief, and shortly he said 'Okay', and the urgent bustle of court preparations continued. We could do no more except wait. I smoothed Bob's hair, and wondered what I looked like and reflected it didn't really matter, Bob was the one who had to look professional, authoritative, I was invisible after all.

The car deposited us on the road at the side of the court buildings and we had to walk round to the front to enter. My legs were a bit wobbly, so it was good to calm them down a bit, give them a bit of a stretch. It was an imposing edifice. Built, I suppose, to unnerve transgressors, its grey, neo-gothic exterior appeared implacably virtuous, everything signalling the importance within. I was nervous enough without this building's looming intimidation. I didn't even find it elegant. *A bit of beauty wouldn't have gone amiss,* my distracted thoughts mumbled.

The hearing

On entering we were almost immediately into a long, grey corridor, virtually a narrow hall. I noticed a series of wide, wood-panelled doors along one side. The corridor was full of chatting groups and importantly scurrying figures in black gowns and greying wigs. Our group too was importantly chatting. It seemed they were trying to find out which judge was allocated to which courtroom and which courtroom our case would be heard in. The BBC's barrister arrived, back from scurrying around, a bit puzzled: the application, it appeared, would be heard by a judge who specialised in property law. They all seemed to think it significant, I couldn't tell why. The wood-panelled doors opened, my stomach lurched, and we headed for our allocated courtroom.

Bob and I sat together at the back on a slightly raised bench directly opposite the judge. *If he looks up he will see us,* I thought. It started abruptly. The Home Office barrister rose. 'We apply for this to be held in camera, as it deals with official secrets...' His words rolled along the quiet air, accompanied by a lopsided declaiming gesture. It was almost Shakespearean, but this wasn't a play we were in. Clutching Bob's shoulder I whispered, 'What does it mean?' 'Shh, just a minute...' The judge was gathering up his documents. 'I will withdraw to consider the application.'

Around us everyone was talking. I began to understand. This was an application for a secret hearing. No-one could watch, report, or indeed refer to it. There were a number of observers and reporters, as well as myself, who would have to leave the courtroom and pretend none of this was happening. If we lost, it meant Bob could give no response. Bob, the men, the work, would be rendered invisible, expunged from any public record, denied any mention, let alone a voice: this, I suddenly realised, was always the fierce intention behind the injunction.

My shaking fatigue was now compounded by an overwhelming anger, Bob's welcoming grasp steadied me somewhat, but it couldn't stop my weary brain filling with unanswerable questions as we sat waiting for the judge to return. *What was this? How could the might of the State be used to suppress discussion in this way? How could a doctor, trying to understand and treat violence, to make it visible, and open for debate, be a danger to the State? Sticking to 'talking head' theory could be safely ignored, but together with the men was it too real? Was it really just about control, control of the message, control of what could and should be seen? What was there to fear?* I thought of the affidavit, so carefully constructed, and wondered whether the judge could see the integrity in it. *If he didn't, would Bob be facing prosecution?*

The courtroom was expectant with quiet mutterings and shuffling. No-one knew how long the judge would be out. It added to our pain. Then the door behind his bench opened, and the judge resumed his seat. Placing the documents in front of him, he looked around the room. Desperate for any friendly clue, I had noticed his wasn't an all-important walk. Of mid-stature, he appeared at ease and confident. 'The application to be heard in camera is denied. We're not dealing with a naval shipyard here.'

The relief from his pronouncement was wonderful, a glimmer of rationality was creeping into the proceedings. I could stay. I looked ahead, hoping the judge might somehow see my support, my steadiness. He was now turning to the Home Office barrister, who rose with a flourish and started on a fluent tale of mayhem if the programme were aired, coupled with a damning indictment of the doctor for breaches of contract, breaches of all manner of confidentialities and for contravening the Official Secrets Act. In sum, for acting illegally and dangerously. The Home Office was acting to protect the prisons, the prisoners, and the general public. He ended dramatically, declaiming, 'We would have no problem if the prisoners' faces were blacked out, and actors spoke their words.'

So that was it! The faces of these men, the voices of these men were the danger that had to be totally erased. The only people who had authentic experience, who could authentically inform, had to be erased. Was everyone just too busy hating and fearing even to attempt to be informed? To understand? It was a complete, persuasive diatribe, given with a bland surety by a man paid to weave plausibility out of scraps of thin air. If any one of the scraps were believed we were doomed. I saw the judge unhurriedly making notes. The affidavit I knew held a total refutation, but would it be enough?

Damage-seeking missiles, cruelly demeaning accusations manufactured especially for us spiralled on and on through the air, piercing my confidence. It was horrible. Bob was upright, intent, listening. He squeezed my hand. His certainty warmed me.

Then it was time for the back-up to proclaim: a smallish man in an ill-fitting suit matching his somewhat uneasy demeanour stood up. It was a prison psychiatrist. Pulling a sheet of paper out of his pocket, he began. He was standing sideways, looking down at the scrap in his hand. It appeared to be a lined foolscap sheet of scrawled handwriting, not even covering the page. He asserted his professional opinion that the programme would cause riots. The men were dangerous. Looking up, the judge enquired politely, 'Do you know who the men are? Have you treated them?'

'No.'

'Have you seen the programme?'

'No.'

A little welcome confidence returned as I thought, *Surely there was no credibility there,* but I remained more than anxious — we had still to absolutely refute all the contractual allegations. The BBC's barrister rose. It was clear he was using Bob's affidavit. Patiently, he went through the narrative of Bob's time at Parkhurst, teasing out the legal points and producing the documents that supported Bob's declaration. Then it was over. The judge retired. We could expect the verdict later that afternoon.

Somehow we found a coffee and a sandwich, and talked to the lawyers, trying for a little hope. No-one would predict. Everyone was edgy.

The judge's ruling

Entering the courtroom once more, I settled into a mood of calming fatalism. The judge began to read his judgement. It was a lengthy, coherent statement which reviewed all the legal issues at each stage. I knew it was going our way when he said, 'Dr Johnson made his intentions clear three years ago asking for your response. Why have you waited until now to act?... Dr Johnson has treated the men over a number of years and has seen the programme, and judges there will be no riots. I am inclined to accept his word.'

And finally, the longed-for verdict: 'The application for an injunction is denied. The programme may be broadcast.'

So that's the end, Bob and I thought, hugging each other with more, so much more than relief. Except that it wasn't. Instead, there was an immediate noisy scurrying.

'What's going on?'

'It's the Home Office barrister, he's asking for leave to appeal.'

'Oh Bob, for heaven's sake...'

Why, why? They'd lost... it was mid-afternoon, I wanted to ring my kids and tell them it was being broadcast... that we'd won, we'd won! Outside, we stood around on the grey, flagged courtyard, this new waiting compounded by a cruelly-destroyed elation. Gazing at the cluster of BBC men and lawyers, I was merely an invisible lurker. Bob was in the circle, but there seemed embarrassment at having him there. The thought hurt. He was an irrelevance, no longer needed now and as impotent as I was. *How long does a bloody appeal take?* I stood, sat, and walked around...

'The judge has just refused leave to appeal.' Rushing up to Bob I said 'Wonderful, can't we just go?' It was around five o'clock by now and there would just be time to get the programme out, and I could have a rest at last. There was scarcely a pause in their mutterings, they appeared to be expecting more. The lawyers especially seemed to be buzzing.

'They're going to appeal the refusal... they're looking for the judges now, they need three.' *Appeal the refusal to appeal?? It's a Russian doll of a farce, how long can they go on? Three? Looking for three judges? The place is stuffed with judges, they don't have to look far!*

And then an offer. 'They will drop the appeal if we tell them who the men are...'

These were weasel words no doubt, and trust was in short supply as the arguments went back and forth. The broadcast was put on hold as the appeal was dangled. It was getting perilously late for the programme to be broadcast that night.

With what reluctance I can only guess, but the capitulation finally came. Unable to find three judges willing to hear their particular appeal they'd had to concede. With half an hour to go, instructions were given to broadcast. We had actually won.

Clutching a bottle of Krug, we took a taxi to Tom Mangold's house. We were going to watch the broadcast together. Bob had promised him the Krug way back in the beginning. Receiving it, Tom was astonished, saying, 'Many promise, but this is the only time I can remember a promise being delivered...' Noticing this little interchange with such a smoothly, worldly-wise man, I knew, as he didn't, that Bob always meant what he said, and did what he promised. It was this integrity that had just seen us through the High Court, and what had endeared me to him all those years ago.

The familiar music announcing *Panorama* came cheerfully waltzing into the room as we settled to watch. Flashing up came the title: 'Predators.' It was a shock. We hadn't seen that this morning, in fact I didn't recall seeing any title. Suddenly my heart, my head, my sense was swamped with worry. I didn't want this exposure of Bob, his work, the men. Conflicted, I also knew it needed to be seen. Even today this *Panorama* music clutches me with a long-gone dread, and I rarely watch it.

It seemed to be a programme of contrasts. Bob and the men, powerful, real and compelling, and the alternative hidden behind careful statistics and blurred faces. It ended with a professor, despite his scepticism, conceding the need for evaluation. 'It deserves to be analysed, maybe he is onto something...' It wasn't joined-up, but just maybe there was an opportunity for the serious evaluation of this unique record of work.

The BBC, forced to make contingency plans, had advertised a non-contentious transport programme. No review copies of 'Predators' had been distributed. There could now be no publicity for this hard-won, unique documentary. We hadn't even had time to inform friends it was going out after all, so many never saw it: they hadn't bothered to watch, not being much interested in transport, and back then the technology only gave them a single shot at viewing it.

Tom, watching with us, was discreetly furious. Whatever else, the lifeblood of investigative journalism was public attention. His was the face of *Panorama*, known for groundbreaking news and hard-hitting, accurate presentation, but this was destined to be stillborn from the screen. Frustrated, he showed us the two-page spread meant to be syndicated out—a rare scoop, a mighty splash, informative, solidly-researched journalese, but now useless, and it wasn't only his thwarted journalese that concerned him: the programme itself had been altered, it was almost *ten minutes shorter* than the one we'd seen earlier that day. The producer was outraged we were told, and had insisted that his name be taken off the credits. Too tired, I failed to fully grasp what this supposed action of his really meant.

It was all too much like 'the curate's egg', good in parts, and our exhaustion was deeply magnified by disappointment. We needed to be home, so instead of birthday jollities we took the late train. I speculated wearily on the perils of colliding with the wishes of a determined Home Secretary. Home Office tactics were already succeeding in neutralising any impact...

Bob looked distinctive, and recognisable, in his suit, with the redoubtable tie still doing its stuff. Glad the carriage was almost empty, I was still nervous. The last, rather belated, attempt by the BBC to help us was a warning: to keep our doors locked. There could be door-steppers around. Would anyone recognise Bob? After all, he had just been seen by a few million people. I realised how much I craved the security of privacy. I patted the reassuringly rough stone of the gatepost as we staggered into our welcoming home. Dropping our bags on the floor, we went upstairs. I wanted a bath. Bob wanted to sleep. Tomorrow was waiting.

CHAPTER 21

After-days...

The telephone was ringing in the far distance. I twitched, half awake. It stopped, then started again. Nudging Bob, I said, 'Should I answer it?' 'It's only eight o'clock, they'll leave a message' he muttered. So began another media flurry, but this time more raucous, more insistent. Other TV outlets, aware of the sensational nature of the footage, pressed for access. My daybook was to fill with requests for interviews, talks, and advice. Letters started to arrive.

Bob brought a cafetière of coffee along with toast, porridge and orange juice on a large round tray, placing it beside me on the bed. 'I suppose we ought to see if there's anything in the *Guardian* about it, though they did say it would only be news if the Home Office had succeeded.' 'Suppose so, I'll get it later.'

We chatted wearily on, trying to make sense of it all, to extract some comforts. Why was the Home Office so intent on suppressing it? It was a 'good news' story surely, an attempt within the Prison Service to make prisoners less dangerous. I reflected on the ire of the Home Secretary, faced with the escape of the three prisoners. It felt similar, but this time it was the prisoners' faces that had escaped, and Bob, not John, deemed culpable.

Tom Mangold must have thought his careful, professional, deeply-researched programme had been arbitrarily ruined, its balance and the meaning destroyed. And for the producer it was, if what we had heard was true, an extreme action to disown a project he had worked on for months, the very opposite of the credit demanded by all working in the industry. Not only had the BBC broken faith with the production team they had broken faith with us and our carefully agreed understanding. Attempting to identify the differences in our two viewings, we recalled a sense of satisfaction and agreement with our first one. It had seemed coherent, and balanced. The second viewing felt uncomfortable, and truncated, but we couldn't really know.

Drinking our welcome morning reviver, I thought inconsequentially how I'd like a set of clean white china mugs, and not this motley collection accreted over the years. *At least I'd have something that was calm and uncluttered.* Still lying in bed gathering our thoughts and energy for the day ahead, we were finding some comfort together. It was a huge relief that Bob had escaped with his professional integrity intact, and at least some of the truth was out there.

Later that morning I collected the *Guardian*. There was an article, not front-page but prominent enough. I always had a friendly chat with the white-haired woman in charge of this tiniest of Post Offices, and she was discreetly aware of some of our doings. On this particular day, as well as 'Good morning', she said 'Oh goodness!' Quickly reading the headline—'Doctor must return jail tapes'—and a Home Office spokesman's comment, confirming that action would be taken regardless of the failed injunction, my recent calm evaporated. Rushing back into our home, I shouted for Bob.

'What's going on?'

'Look, look what it says here!'

Soberly, we sat down and scrutinised the article line-by-line. It was groundless nonsense, and also frighteningly feasible. The Home Affairs editor of the *Guardian* had contacted the Home Office, and deduced they were preparing for legal action unless the tapes were returned or wiped clean. The Home Office were intent on using the Official Secrets Act and the catch-all 'duty of confidentiality to the Crown.' They were demanding the names of those who had seen their content.

What a cruel, unthinking contempt! A contempt so utter it first ignored the work, then destroyed the place of its creation, and finally demanded total destruction of any evidence it ever took place. *What a book-burning was this! Despite a total ignorance of the content, the actual hard-won therapy, that was nevertheless what they wanted destroyed.* No material trace could be left behind.

Sitting together at our old kitchen table all those years ago, that was the astounding intention we were experiencing. Bob had clearly rattled some monster, in some cage!

I banged around the kitchen, clearing away pots and scrubbing a neglected sink. I was fearful, but more than that, I was angry.

What was so bloody wrong with trying to make dangerous people less dangerous? What was so bloody wrong in showing how it can happen? What was so bloody wrong in letting dangerous people talk about how they became dangerous? What was so bloody wrong in letting them talk about changing? What was so bloody wrong in seeing their faces? In seeing the actual living challenge, the disaster that needs solving? What was so bloody wrong in showing the actual living reality of problems society has to confront if it's ever going to solve them? So what to do now?

Anger fuelled our energy, and Bob penned a letter that appeared in the *Guardian* the following day. He threw down his gauntlet aiming directly at the ideology of the Home Secretary.

'He now threatens me, unless I destroy my 700 hours of videotapes, something I will never do... healthy minds and stable societies can't exist without truth, trust, and consent... can we not lift our minds above kindergarten squabbles...?'

It was lunchtime. Unusually, Bob didn't feel like much either, so we took yet more coffee and some biscuits into the garden where we sat in some early spring sunshine.

'The snowdrops are coming up', I said. 'They always do around my birthday.'

'It's not been much of a birthday for you.'

'No, not exactly a barrel of laughs. Do you think Howard means it?'

'Absolutely. Look what he said about John. Look how he treated Derek Lewis. Look what he says—Okay, okay, so—worst case—fight it, lose, go to prison...'

Bob laughed, and so started the most surreal of all our debates.

'It would be an interesting experience, I could do a lot of writing...'

'No, I think it'd be better if I went inside, the women's prisons might be easier...'

But for us, there was worse to consider, and to prevent. Using my own hinterland of friendship and support, I passed the tapes into the respectful hands of those I trusted. Bob knew only that they were gone. I knew only that I had handed them over, and neither of us knew where they were. It felt like a wartime mission to hide secrets from the enemy. Faced with a barrage of questions and letters, the Prison Service issued a press release stating, 'It was wrong of Dr Johnson to claim he did any good.' This was professional assassination; this was unadorned libel. Swiftly my lawyer niece penned an incisive letter and a retraction was quickly issued. Sadly, the PR machine had been unguardedly revealing doing good was never ever on the prison menu.

Social scientists, criminologists, therapists and their organizations began requesting interviews, seeking research and offering collaboration. The vision was entrancing: established centres for research, and the treatment of psychopathic distress, floated into my mind. Any possibility of collaboration was to evaporate as soon as an awareness of the legal threats emerged. The tapes were becoming toxic, as toxic as Bob, untouchable, unusable, unmentionable. So too was the *Panorama* programme. Even today I search the BBC archives in vain.

Persistent requests from Bob to follow up his patients, to find out where they were, to write to them were all ignored, and it was only slowly that we began to hear anything. The inelegant, scrawled scrap of a letter lay on the table between us, name and prisoner number on the outside of the envelope, as per regulations.

'Their solicitor fellow came round, wanted us to sue you…course we had nowt to do with it. You must have made a lot of enemies, they had it in for me…'

Final meeting

It was a time of glorious summer sun and breeze as we set off, heading into the wind for an afternoon of sailing with John. He'd recovered some of his old zip, along with a new berth as a mental health manager on the island. Released from the strictures of Prison Service employment, he had written an excoriating attack on events surrounding his removal. Sitting in the cockpit with my back to the bulkhead, I was happily watching them. John was at the helm, Bob winching in the ropes, we were going fast, scudding over the white caps of the waves, breezy salt spray starting to drench me. John was laughing as he shook the spray off his glasses when Bob shouts, 'Change course we're heading for the buoy!'

It's always a bit tricky if a boat heels over, and the sails are in the way of actually seeing where you're heading. Some boats, I later noticed, have a transparent section in the main sail. John didn't have this luxury, and relied on his confident knowledge, and his crew. The crew kept shouting. John began shouting. I crouched down out of the noisy cracking flapping busyness, and noticed the enormous buoy speeding past us. 'We have just missed…'

I handed up the coffee to a waiting Bob and John, and settled back into my seat against the bulkhead where I could see the wake of the boat, and the distance we had travelled. How could I have known this was the last time we were to chat together? John was vibrant, strong, chatty, seductive even. Snatches of the old exhilaration emerged as new ideas were tossed around. Some absurd, some more real. I wondered what power John really had in this new job of his. A surface zip was there but to what depth I couldn't tell. I sensed a hollowing out as though his self was more bravado than belief.

And Bob, well, he hadn't had such status or role to lose, only his dreams, and his quest, and the men had given him the success he strove for. His anger, and his sadness was because they'd taken his patients away from him. And me, what of me? Recalling that last momentary meeting of these two minds, alive with jostling possibilities, my heart clutched in a sorrow of 'what could have beens.'

Farewell

Tenderly those who loved John laid him to rest on the edge of a cornfield overlooking the sea. My husband's last assistance to him was to untangle the ropes, so that his descent into his grave of red dry earth was smooth and quiet. The sadness and love that descended with him was stronger than the ropes; quietly we dropped red earth on his coffin as we held him in our hearts. With heartbreaking irony, this bouncy humanitarian and former Number One Governor of Parkhurst Prison was now the number one and sole occupant of a tiny newly-consecrated parish cemetery, at the bottom of the downs and a short walk from his old stone house.

His death of a sudden massive heart attack aged 51 was shocking. The *Independent* in its obituary referred to the extreme censure John received at the time of the Parkhurst escapes commenting, 'And so a man hitherto almost universally regarded as conscientious, caring, thoughtful and committed, found himself to be in the eye of the storm, or at least a House of Commons debate.' John was a vulnerable man who wore his heart on his sleeve. A civil servant not allowed to speak out, he was a humanitarian who was finally betrayed by the Prison Service and the system for which he worked so hard.

The tiny church and churchyard filled to overflowing as hundreds arrived. I saw many from the Prison Service: governors, civil servants, officers, all sad, grim-faced, regretful. They were to organize their own memorial service later, but for the moment were they wondering, *A scapegoat too far?* All knew the truth: an impossible job, with a denial of resources. One escape too far for the political safety of the Home Secretary, but gagged by contract, the Official Secrets Act, fear and wishful thinking, there was little action taken to save John. He resigned, halved his salary, and it broke his heart.

Bob and I lingered in the graveyard before walking down the hill to John's old home for a glass of the 'decent red wine' that he'd specified for his funeral. His wife had asked for flowers, and they were there in aching abundance, a double row almost the breadth of the cemetery, bringing the sadness and regrets of prisons and prisoners from all over the country. She was to distribute these around the island to every mental health centre. A painful and generous task in honour of John and his last role.

CHAPTER 22

After-shocks

One: The Big Man

I am looking out at the sea once more. It's summer and the sunlight is revealing the lines of brown sandbanks hiding beneath the waiting waves as they gently move to the shore, catching the unwary perhaps. The telephone rings competing with the quiet of the garden. I go inside.

'It's E!' shouts a loud male voice down the line as though unused to being heard. I detect the echoing bustle of an institution in the background. 'What's the weather like on the Isle of Wight?' he goes on conversationally, 'It's a bit too warm in here.'

'It's fine here', I say, 'there's a breeze from the sea.'

'That's nice', he says, and I know he means it. 'Sue...'

'Yeah...'

'Will you tell Dr Bob to stop trying to get me out of here. I am doing fine.'

'Okay.' I paused a fraction. 'Yes, I will. Take care...'

'Okay, Sue. Gotta go now. Cheerio.'

This big man was the first prisoner to accept Bob's challenge all those years ago. The transcripts of his interviews so freely and generously given show his agonising insight. I sat down, suddenly feeling sick. This man was approaching seventy-years-of-age. He knew Bob would never give up on him. He also knew Bob's efforts were futile and possibly destabilising. He was facing a reality that Bob himself didn't want to see. He had now decided to accommodate himself to the facts of his situation and to remain incarcerated for the rest of his life.

Two: Baby of the wing

The doors on the far side of the hall opened and a group of prisoners shuffled in. I had noticed that in prisons they always seemed to shuffle, small slow dreary steps. I suppose time is all there remains to negotiate, and small steps fill it better and large, brisk purposive prancing isn't useful currency.

So, everyone was stunned when one of the men actually ran. Racing across the room, delightedly bellowing, 'My psychiatrist's wife!' and throwing his arms around me, he grabbed me in a huge hug. He was grinning widely, and I recognised the long-gone figure of that oh-so-young man I'd met in Parkhurst. He'd filled out a bit, was a man. No longer young, he seemed confident, jovial, sociable. The watching men were curious and baffled.

'When did you have a psychiatrist?' one shouted.

His instant reply was proud, 'In C-Wing, Parkhurst.'

'You can't have been...'

'Yes, I was.'

He replied almost happily, I thought, but I detected a perceptible shrinking away in the men. C-Wing was a horror story, and they were a self-selected group who wanted just to talk quietly with some volunteer visitors. It didn't include the notoriously mad and violent, in their minds. It wasn't making sense to anyone there as S was affable, and clearly liked.

S had an eager, determined purpose. This was his chance. 'Tell Bob I didn't mean to hit him... I hope he's forgiven me.' *How many years had he been waiting to say that?* Sadness nearly overwhelmed me as his big eager smile displayed such relief, the end of waiting, of worrying. I wanted, I needed to reassure him. 'It's okay... Bob told me all about it, he said it was his own fault, he should have noticed what you were like. There's nothing to forgive. He'll be excited I met you. He'll want to know how you've been getting on. It's really okay.'

This was his present to Bob, his chance of longed-for reconnection. It was a powerful statement, a demonstration of the lasting truth of Bob's work, and for me it was enormous, an unsought gift. Even if this was all I got to see of the men, it couldn't ever have been wasted time. S talked non-stop, he was a bursting dam. There was so much he wanted to say, wanted to know. We were in a bubble, and I scarcely noticed the visitors, or the twenty or so prisoners exchanging carefully constrained glances and conversations around us. We sat and talked until the allotted hour was up.

It was of course against all protocols, this delighted connection. The warnings had been severe: don't give personal details, handshakes only, dress discreetly, prisoners can be manipulative. Only later did I wonder why the officers didn't approach: 'Break it up now you know the rules.' I can see now how no-one dared destroy what they were witnessing.

The volunteers, normally quite chatty after such visits, scarcely found words, and I, well I just wanted to see Bob and tell him. *What a title! What an accolade he'd given me, what precious meaning it had for him! I realised I had always had a job. I was indeed his prison psychiatrist's wife. I was never really invisible, an ignored observer, I had always been immersed in shaping what was to come.* All those years ago the man in the blue jumper had known this, and now I'd come full circle with a strangely similar appeal for help. This time it wasn't 'Will you let him come?' but 'Tell him I hope he's forgiven me.'

It was Bob's time to wait for me, for the door to open. He was as surprised as I'd been. 'Oh Bob, he's been worrying for years, he said tell Bob I didn't mean to hit him, I hope he's forgiven me. I nearly cried. I said you'd told me all about it, that it was your fault.'

'How wonderful you saw him! We couldn't ever have predicted that. I'd backed him into a corner, he knew no other way to stop me. Really great you went, and could tell him it was okay, I never got the chance...' There was a sadness in his voice, coming from an old outrage I felt would never really go away. He'd been prevented from seeing his patients. I could understand S's fearful hitting out. *But Bob's colleagues, what had they to fear from an excess of humanity?* My sadness matched, and merged, with his...

Three: The man in the blue jumper

It was a tricky journey by train. The Home Office crib-sheet accompanying the visiting order had identified the nearest train station and proffered a map of sorts; it was a small bleak little station, stopping trains were rare, visiting slots rarer. It meant a wait, anyway, and I'd chosen HM waiting room for the purpose after the mile-and-a-half trek from the station.

I suddenly felt overwhelmed with discomfort. *Maybe the station would have been better, at least it hasn't rained.* I'd been careful with my clothes, they were discreetly quiet, non-committal, I had thought, but here, set against the clothing of the other waiting women, they oozed privilege, comfort, class, an educated authority. The watching officers noticed. It didn't compute, I wasn't part of their thinking about the generality of scum going through to meet scum. I was no longer invisible. I offended their need to know everything. I could hear them thinking, *What is she? Not down as a visiting legal... psychology we know... maybe one of those religious do-gooders.* Then one stalked over.

'How do you know him?' he said.

'How indeed?' A question awaiting a lifetime of answers. My mind flashed back — to the man in the blue jumper's question, and my unspoken response.

'At Parkhurst', I said. The name still registered, despite no longer existing.

'On the chaplaincy team then are you?'

'No', I said, with an angry delight in their bafflement as I proceeded through a security that felt so very intrusive. *No pens, no pencils, no bags, nothing but a bit of cash for the vending machine.*

Entering the large visiting room, I saw small tables and chairs bolted in place around it. The mainly women visiting, familiar with the procedures, selected tables and sat down. I followed. The tables weren't all inhabited, and I found one without neighbours. A door at the far end opened and the room became awash with chatter as the men, spotting their visitors, sat down. *A strange sort of party game without the music.* He saw me and came across. I stood and he shook my hand.

'Hello Sue', he said, 'Would you like a drink?'

'Thanks, what do we do?'

'There's a machine over there and we can get biscuits.'

'Right... I've got some pounds, they said I'd need them.'

It was a sad little dance, we were breaking the ice, finding something to do. I was shocked by his appearance and he knew it. He was wearing a jacket and ill-fitting trousers, clutching at a dignity the place was stripping from him. Sipping the horrible coffee I said, 'How are you?'

'I've got diabetes now... it's the drugs I think, but I can't stop them. Just get banged-up if I refuse.'

I detected a slight tremor in the hand that grasped his biscuit, another of the drugs' side-effects. I winced, this was awful. Longing for another reality, I said, 'Do you remember that first meeting you were wearing a blue jumper?' I'd made a terrible mistake. The memory, the thought, the idea...

'I don't like you to see me like this.' He was still clever, acutely aware, but this time an awareness that was too much. He stood and said, 'I'm sorry I need a cigarette, I can only smoke outside.'

I watched him leave. It was too much for me too, I think he knew that.

An ending

I am on my erratically daily walk up the hill. Early sun has cast its shimmering light over a calmly undulating sea. As I climb higher, rare frost sparkles in delight. I gently touch a Gingko tree, apparently a tough, slow-growing survivor from the time when dinosaurs nibbled its scalloped leaves. Now these leaves are sheltering a cherished memory: a small name label which says simply 'Remembering', the date 1991.

Nineteen-ninety-one was the year I first went through the gates of Parkhurst Prison, and yesterday, so many years after he'd pushed his grimly empty chair out through the gates and into another life, Bob had entered those gates once more, to assess a prisoner deemed too nasty to be released. This time he entered not with the laughing encouragement of a benign Governor but to fulfil a legal request for a Parole Board report. Standing at the door I had given him a suddenly anxious hug, ruffling his now thinner, greying hair and said banally, 'Good luck', and then later, anxiously, 'How did you get on?' and 'Were you laying ghosts?' He'd smiled and said, 'There were no ghosts to lay.'

How could he be so sure? Mine were still there. The man he saw had displayed the same characteristics of those long gone C-Wing boys. Where were they all now? A snatch of a nostalgic song moves into my head...

Where have all the young men gone?
Long time passing...
They've gone to graveyards everyone,
When will they ever learn?

My thoughts were brutal: *They are in graveyards of the soul, every one*, and it was with relief I had heard Bob's cheerful voice on his return. 'It's clearer than ever. He really got what I was saying. I think I can help... but listen to this, he'd been told "Johnson used to work here... never did much. You won't get anything out of seeing him. He's only in it for the money".'

Shocked and angry I wanted to hear Bob defend himself.

'What did you say?'

'I didn't say anything, I just laughed. It shows I had an impact!'

How had this lingered, some folk tale passed down through the culture of the very building? The old name itself was long gone, the men dispersed, and a new HMP Isle of Wight had arisen from closures, mergers, cuts and redundancies. Old familiar worries I had thought inactive clutched at my stomach. *Never did much!!* I was furious, impotently angry. *Of course it hadn't lingered, it had stuck, it had festered.* The laughing confident optimistic figures of a so-young John and Bob came floating into my vision, dancing figures as they pranced, chatting animatedly, down to the sea, such sparkling chunks of light, illuminating the dungeons with hope, with possibilities and kindness.

Back from my walk I listen to the strains of Schubert echoing through our home. Lying on our new extra-large and extra comfy bed, and gazing out to sea, I have kept the door open. The music is gentle, complex, lyrical but Bob no longer plays on his own, he has a companion. John's cherished step-daughter is playing those magnificent duets. Hoots of delighted laughter fill the air.

Epilogue

So, there it is. I gently lay down the pages of another read-through of what? Of memory, of feeling, of thoughts? My reading glasses are stronger now, I keep them on hand tied to a yellow cord around my neck. That was a slice of long-gone time, a precious period of now fossilised experience, when our energy, our idealism was briefly given rein, and the possibilities of optimism and of change were grasped. The world could have turned a lovely way up. I have a nearly-contented accommodation to this history of ours.

*****

Pushing the door wide I saw the heap of assorted letters that had obstructed its smooth opening, and turned to help Bob in. I had taken a wheelchair to the ferry, being anxious that it was all going to be too much for him. Uneasy, I hadn't wanted him to leave the hospital quite so soon after the operation. I could tell he was still high from the drugs. We'd waited for a taxi with an accompanying nurse, and his normal over-the-top banter was veering into nonsense. I could see she too was thinking it might be too soon, but Bob was adamant, and so we had made the crossing and now were finally and thankfully home.

The garden gate no longer clanged. It was a new one made out of old oak beams we had salvaged from the demolition of Ladysmith Barracks in Lancashire all those years ago. It didn't exactly fit too well, and needed a strong shove, but I loved its oldness, and the way it shut out passing gazes.

Now we could rest. Ludicrously, I was still using a crutch, a legacy from a broken pelvis which had meant Bob's operation had been delayed. The relief to be back, together, and seemingly okay was immense. I put the kettle on, still lime green, but now a sleeker version of its long-gone self. Retro stylish, it was a recent addition and thoughtful present. We hugged each other, almost, I recall, in the same place we'd hugged all those years ago when I saw myself in the mirror and felt such a piercing awareness of the journey ahead. The mirror was still there, but this time our hugs were brief, almost perfunctory, a reassuring acknowledgement of being safely home.

'You okay?' I said, suddenly enormously weary. Bob was rifling through the post, still jovially rambling in a demob-happy way. And then: 'What's this?'

Puzzled, he waved a large brown envelope with 'GMC' on it. The General Medical Council is the regulatory body for doctors. Bob paid annual fees to be retained on their register, and had recently undergone mandatory appraisal and revalidation. All had been well, and indeed the process, bureaucratic though it was, had given him some glowing encouragement for the work he did. Unconcerned, I imagined this was merely some more self-congratulatory PR bumph.

'It's a complaint. I am a danger to the public and my patients.'

'What?! Let me see.'

'It's not you, it's a mistake, they say here you work at Wakefield Prison.'

But it wasn't a mistake. A consultant forensic psychiatrist Bob had met briefly at a Parole Board tribunal was in deadly earnest. He'd taken angry and destructive exception to Bob's report on a prisoner. So, the investigation began, and we plunged into a made-up world where words are brutal objects, rinsed of all connection to living meaning. This time they were missiles cruelly, deliberately shaped to destroy that living target, Bob. A calculated, invisible expression of anger. 'You pissed them off', said the barrister, used to observing the rage behind actions.

Pre-invented words were waiting for their moment of destructive glory. A justification for all the efforts of committee after committee, producing report after report. So many years ago now, Bob talked of fear as 'the master emotion.' Behind every anger there was fear.

The peril was never the prisoners nor the officers nor even the colossus of the Prison Service and the Home Office. No, the lurking danger was ever the hatred of colleagues, the implacable bureaucratic might of the GMC their weapon. Could this actually be final destruction? Already my hurt seemed of a different order. Snatches of song come to me: *You don't know what you've got 'til it's gone, They paved paradise and put up a parking lot.* And what a 'parking lot' ... labyrinthine, costly, its entry cruel but its exit invisible.

Just as I had used the garden, the sea, the sky as a piercingly beautiful solace to my worries back in those 'dungeon days' as I now called our time at Parkhurst, so Bob was to disappear into the brambles at the extremity of the garden, and he began creating a wood-and-glass haven, away from the questions, the emails, the conversations, the threats, the usual cruelty.

I hear my breath, a hugely painful, seeping sigh, an unbidden and pristine hurt, freshly minted just for me. *I can't pause this living moment, and steal backwards to a time of gentle calm. There is stuff, so much stuff, to do. Documents, protocols, guidelines, growing in extent and circularity. Angels on the head of a pin. All assuming, indeed mandating, their own brand of absolutely certain knowledge of the human condition.* I think of the valiant efforts of thinkers and philosophers down the centuries, searching for this holiest of grails. *How would they have tackled this oh-so-unkind arrogant absurdity? And now, how indeed would we?*

My newly strengthened glasses have work ahead.

Milton Keynes UK
Ingram Content Group UK Ltd.
UKHW040123290324
440304UK00003B/30

9 781914 603303